Rebalance Your Vagus Nerve Superhighway:

The Ultimate 3-Step Strategic Roadmap to Relieve Pain, Calm Your Mind, Improve Sleep, and Restore Gut Health

Dr. Kerri L. Jones, N.M.D.

ISBN 978-1-968147-01-3 Paperback

Contents

Dedication

Wow! The glory goes to God! I want to thank Him for the many gifts He has given me and the many talents- the gift of being a healer, a way with words, and a creative brain. My life has not been without overwhelming challenges, but I've become stronger, more resilient, and grown closer to Him.

You wouldn't be reading this if my wonderful husband had not believed in me, my desire to educate people about natural, holistic medicine, and my overwhelming need to share what I have learned in medicine and health care with the masses over several decades. Naturopathic Medicine is my passion! He sees me light up and become so alive whenever I talk to anyone about natural medicine.

Despite feeling horrible most days, living with unrelenting, chronic pain, and a rare genetic connective tissue disorder, hypermobile Ehlers-Danlos Syndrome (hEDS), and all of the symptoms and conditions that come along on the daily rollercoaster ride-he supports me 100% in starting this new career of writing and publishing. I could not have done this without you believing in me and agreeing for us to invest in me. David, you are indeed the one God chose for me. He brought us together at this stage in our lives when we both thought we would spend the rest of our lives single. Well, I'm so glad I have you to hold my hand and walk beside me through whatever the Lord has in store for us in the future. I know that no matter whether it is sunshine or storms, the Lord will be with us and continue to watch over and bless us. I love you so much, David; thank you for loving me and my quirky, geeky, and neurodiverse personality. I am blessed beyond measure!

Always, Kerri

Introduction

As a naturopathic medical doctor, I've witnessed countless patients struggling with complex medical issues like chronic pain, anxiety, depression, and a host of other physical and emotional challenges. Almost all of them felt lost, frustrated, and hopeless, bouncing from one specialist to another without finding answers or lasting relief. I understand their frustration and pain intimately, as I, too, continue to face my health battles, including a rare genetic connective tissue disorder called Ehlers-Danlos Syndrome (EDS) and its dozens of related symptoms and conditions.

Through my journey, spanning decades of healthcare work and numerous years of medical practice, I discovered a powerful key to unlocking better health and well-being: the vagus nerve. This remarkable nerve is often overlooked and misunderstood by traditionally trained doctors. The vagus nerve is crucial in regulating the nervous system, emotions, and physical health. When I began to focus on rebalancing my vagus nerve, I experienced profound improvements in my physical and mental/emotional symptoms and overall quality of life.

Imagine your nervous system as a major metropolitan superhighway system, with the vagus nerve as the main highway connecting your brain and body. This highway system has many branches, each leading to different organs and systems carrying vital information through tiny electrical impulses. When traffic flows smoothly, your body functions optimally, and you feel balanced and healthy. But when accidents, roadblocks, or construction slow-downs occur, your health usually suffers, leading to a wide range of symptoms and disorders.

In this book, I invite you to join me on a transformative journey to understand, assess, and optimize your vagus nerve function. We'll delve into the science behind this remarkable nerve, its role in the parasympathetic nervous system, and how it impacts various aspects of your health, including mood, stress levels, digestion, and sleep patterns.

We'll explore the latest research on neuroplasticity (the ability of your brain to form and reorganize its connections, especially in response to learning and experience), Polyvagal Theory (that emphasizes the role of the vagus nerve in your nervous system and the role it plays in regulating our behaviors and overall health) and heart rate variability (the difference in time between your heartbeats), empowering you with the knowledge and tools to take control of your health. You'll discover practical exercises, techniques, and strategies to strengthen your vagus nerve, reduce pain, stress, depression, and anxiety, improve sleep and digestion to promote overall well-being and address many other conditions, including those associated with trauma.

Through a simple three-step process, you'll learn how to:

1. Discover the Science Behind Your Nervous System's Function

2. Assess Your Vagus Nerve Power

3. Rebalance and Optimize Your Vagus Nerve

As we navigate this journey together, I'll share personal stories and insights from my experiences as a patient and a healthcare provider. My goal is to create a caring, supportive, empathetic, and vulnerable space where you don't feel dismissed but feel understood, validated, and inspired to take charge of your health. Whether you're struggling with chronic pain or emotional issues or simply seeking to optimize your well-being, this book is your guide to rebalance and harness the power of your vagus nerve. With curiosity, commitment, and an open mind, you can revitalize your nervous system, build resilience, and experience profound healing. So, one page at a time, let's explore the wonders of the vagus nerve and unlock the keys to a healthier, more balanced life. Your path to wellness starts here, and I'm honored to be your guide.

STEP ONE

Discover The Science Behind Your Nervous System's Function

Chapter 1: Our Journey Begins, Your Nervous System Explained

Years ago, I sat in a small exam room across from a patient, feeling increasingly disconnected from her own body. She described a cascade of symptoms-persistent fatigue, headache, digestive issues, worry, and a lingering sense of dread that she couldn't quite shake. She had seen numerous health professionals in various specialties, each trying to offer her a piece of the puzzle. The pieces never seemed to fit to give her the whole picture. Her story mirrored my own struggles, as I, too, had wandered through the maze of healthcare, seeking answers that seemed elusive.

As I mentioned, years ago, during my personal and professional explorations, I stumbled upon the remarkable and powerful vagus nerve, which shifted my understanding of health and healing. The vagus nerve is part of a vast superhighway system, our nervous system, that governs our body's most fundamental processes and holds the potential to transform not just symptoms but the very fabric of our well-being.

In this chapter, we'll explore the structure and function of the nervous system, the role of the vagus nerve, and how it affects both physical and emotional well-being. Through clear explanations and analogies, you'll gain insight into how the body's communication networks influence your health and discover strategies to support these vital systems.

The vagus nerve acts as a vital communication highway within the nervous system, linking the brain with organs throughout the body. It's like the main artery of the superhighway system, where signals-much like vehicles-move continuously, carrying essential information. Yet, unlike a typical highway, this system is not just about speed and efficiency but also balance and harmony. When the system functions well, signals travel smoothly, ensuring that your heart beats steadily, your digestion operates like clockwork, and your mind feels calm and centered. However, when traffic jams or other traffic issues arise-in the form of stress, trauma, or illness-the flow of information becomes disrupted, resulting in chaos that manifests as physical and emotional symptoms.

Before we explore the vagus nerve's remarkable powers, it's crucial to understand the broader landscape of your nervous system. Imagine it again as an elaborate superhighway system with various highways, lanes, and exits, all working together to keep traffic flowing smoothly. This complex system has two main parts: the central nervous system (CNS) and the peripheral nervous system (PNS). Each plays a unique role, but they are intertwined in a beautiful dance of communication and coordination that keeps your body functioning harmoniously.

Let's take a moment to examine the picture and diagram below. Please don't get overwhelmed by this; it will become more understandable as you read and learn more. As you go through this chapter, refer to this so that you can become more familiar with the different components of your nervous system. Understanding the various parts of your body will make it easier to know how our bodies work and how they become stronger or weaker depending upon your internal and external environment.

NOTE TO READERS: To explain the complex anatomy and physiology of the nervous system and the vagus nerve, I have condensed and simplified the information for your understanding, using analogies to clarify the concepts. I have tried my best to present this information clearly and understandably. If you are a medical or healthcare professional, please note that I have omitted details for the general public. To the general public: You should be able to embark on a journey to understand the human body, its general functioning, and how this function impacts your everyday life. Some of you may be intrigued by this and want to dig deeper to understand the intricate details that medical and healthcare professionals find amazing.

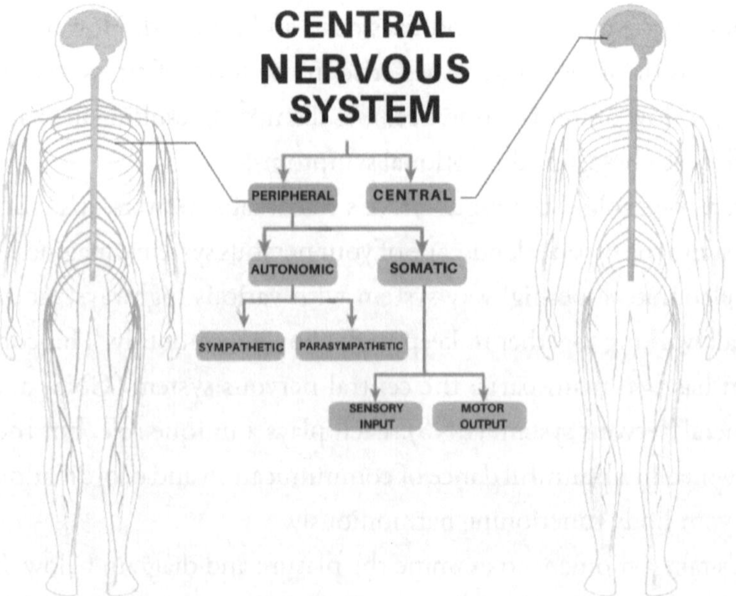

1.1 The Central Nervous System (CNS): The Command Center

The CNS is the mastermind behind all bodily functions. It consists of the brain and spinal cord, which act like the control hub of an advanced traffic system, managing and directing the flow of information. Think of it as the central control room in a high-tech train system, where engineers oversee every schedule with precise timing.

- Brain: The brain is like a super-computer, processing information, making decisions, and generating thoughts, emotions, and memories. It regulates conscious actions, like deciding to lift your arm, and subconscious activities, like maintaining your balance. It is like the mastermind that interprets sensory input (like sight, sound, and touch) and sends out motor instructions to respond appropriately.

- Spinal Cord: It acts as the main cable, efficiently transferring messages between the brain and the rest of the body. It also handles quick reflexes, like pulling your hand away from a hot stove before you even realize it's hot. It's the shortcut road that bypasses lengthy decision-making, allowing you to react quickly to danger.

Example: Imagine accidentally touching a hot pan. Instantly, sensory nerves in your skin detect the intense heat and send a signal through your spinal cord to your brain. Your brain quickly interprets this as pain and sends a message back down through motor nerves to the muscles in your hand. In a split second, your muscles react by pulling your hand away from the danger. This rapid back-and-forth communication between your nerves, spinal cord, and brain helps protect you from getting seriously burned-demonstrating just how fast and efficient your nervous system is.

1.2 The Peripheral Nervous System (PNS): The Information Highway

While the CNS is the command center, the PNS serves as the information highway, a network of roads connecting it to the rest of the body. It acts like a vast interstate system, branching out to every city and neighborhood, ensuring communication between the brain, spinal cord, limbs, and organs.

The PNS is further divided into two systems:

A. Somatic Nervous System (SNS)

B. Autonomic Nervous System (ANS)

A. THE SOMATIC NERVOUS SYSTEM (SNS): THE VOLUNTARY MOVER

The SNS governs all voluntary movements, allowing you to consciously control actions like walking, talking, or waving to a friend. It's like the manual steering system in a car, giving you complete control over where and how you move.

- Motor Neurons carry signals from your brain to your muscles, enabling movement. For example, when you decide to lift your coffee mug, motor neurons send a message from your brain to the muscles in your arm and hand.
- Sensory Neurons: These send information from your senses (like touch, sight, and sound) back to your brain. If you accidentally touch a prickly cactus, sensory neurons in your fingers send a pain signal to your brain, which decides how to respond.

Example: If you decide to take a step forward, the SNS sends a message from your brain to the muscles in your legs, coordinating each movement to maintain balance and stride-using both motor and sensory neurons. It's like choreographing a dance, ensuring every muscle moves in harmony.

B. AUTONOMIC NERVOUS SYSTEM (ANS): THE INVOLUNTARY REGULATOR

The ANS controls automatic bodily functions that occur without conscious thought, such as your heartbeat, digestion, and breathing. It's the autopilot system, keeping you alive and well while you focus on other things.

The ANS has two main branches:

1. **Sympathetic Nervous System (SNS): The Accelerator**
2. **Parasympathetic Nervous System (PNS): The Brake**

Sympathetic Nervous System (SNS): The Accelerator

The Sympathetic Nervous System is your body's "fight or flight" system, designed to protect you in dangerous situations. It prepares you to face the threat or run away by increasing your heart rate, releasing adrenaline (epinephrine), and directing blood flow to your muscles. Think of it as the gas pedal in a car, revving up your system to respond to stress or danger.

Example: If a dog suddenly runs toward you, your sympathetic nervous system kicks in, increasing your heart rate, quickening your breathing, and tensing your muscles so you can run or defend yourself.

Parasympathetic Nervous System (PNS): The Brake

The Parasympathetic Nervous System is the part that allows you to "rest and digest." It calms the body after a stressful event, slowing your heart rate, stimulating digestion, and promoting relaxation. It's like the brake pedal in a car, easing you back into a state of calm and balance.

Example: After escaping the barking dog, your parasympathetic system helps you catch your breath, relaxes your muscles, and returns your heart rate to normal. It's the soothing voice saying, "You're safe now."

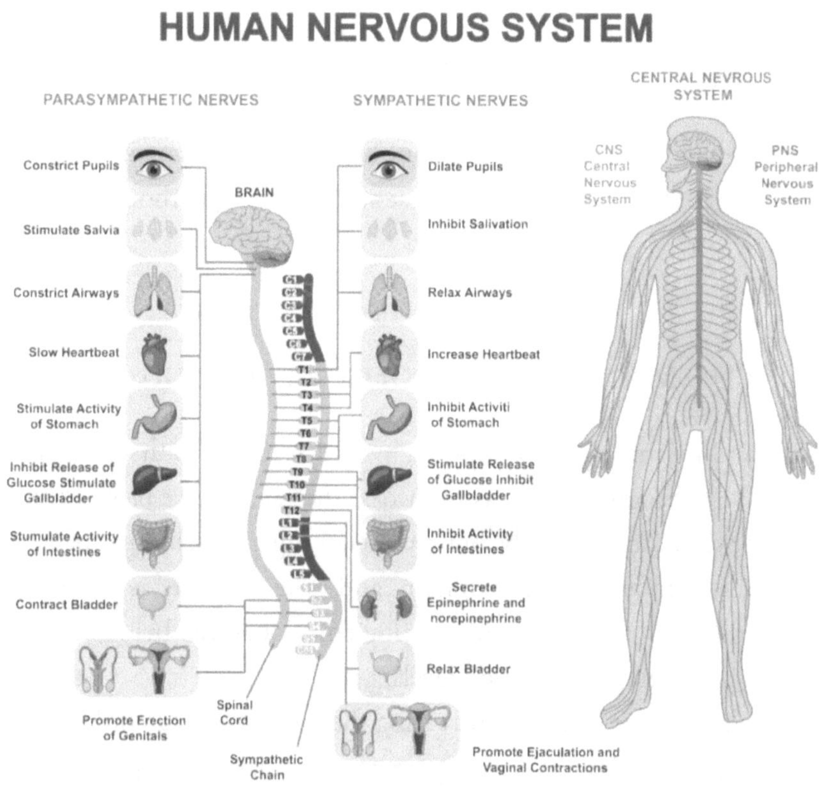

1.3 Bringing It All Together: A Symphony of Balance

The Picture above shows us that CNS and PNS don't work in isolation-they constantly communicate to maintain homeostasis, the body's state of balance. Imagine a well-coordinated orchestra where every instrument (or body part) plays in harmony under the direction of a skilled conductor, much like the central nervous system (CNS). The PNS delivers the music sheets (signals) and ensures every section plays its part perfectly.

- The CNS conducts the overall performance and makes high-level decisions.
- The SNS executes voluntary movements with precision and control.
- The ANS keeps the background rhythm steady, maintaining essential functions like heartbeat and breathing without conscious effort.

WHY THIS MATTERS: THE ROLE OF THE VAGUS NERVE

Understanding this intricate superhighway system is the first step in reclaiming your health. In this vast network, the vagus nerve plays a crucial role as a bridge, connecting the brain to major organs, including the heart, lungs, liver, kidneys, digestive system, and others. It acts as a mediator between the body and mind, influencing emotional well-being, immune function, and even inflammation levels.

This book will explore how nurturing the vagus nerve can unlock healing and transformation. By learning how to stimulate and support this vital nerve, you'll discover a pathway to improved health, emotional balance, and overall vitality.

In the chapters ahead, we'll dive deeper into how vagus nerve function affects four vital areas of your health:

- **Mental and emotional well-being**-including anxiety, depression, trauma, and stress resilience.
- **Chronic pain and inflammation**-and the vagus nerve's role in modulating both.
- **Digestive health**-with a focus on conditions like IBS, bloating, and motility issues.
- **Sleep regulation**-including how vagus nerve tone can impact your ability to fall and stay asleep.

This book will explore how nurturing the vagus nerve can unlock healing and transformation. By learning how to stimulate and support this vital nerve, you'll discover a pathway to improved health, emotional balance, and overall vitality. Together, we'll embark on a journey to rebalance your nervous system, empowering you to live a healthier, happier, and more harmonious life.

1.4 The Cranial Nerves: Express Lanes of the Nervous System

Imagine again the nervous system as an intricate superhighway, where every lane, exit, sign, and intersection plays a vital role in transporting signals throughout the body. The cranial nerves are at the center of this vast communication network—twelve pairs of highly specialized pathways that emerge directly from the brain. These nerves function like express lanes, providing rapid and direct connections between the brain and specific regions of the head, neck, and even some organs in the body.

Each cranial nerve has a unique function, like different service roads in a city, each leading to specific neighborhoods to manage essential operations. These nerves exist in pairs, one serving the right side of the body and the other the left, ensuring symmetrical communication and function. They are responsible for a variety of critical tasks, including sensory perception (such as sight, smell, and taste), motor control (like eye movement and facial expressions), and autonomic functions (such as heart rate and digestion).

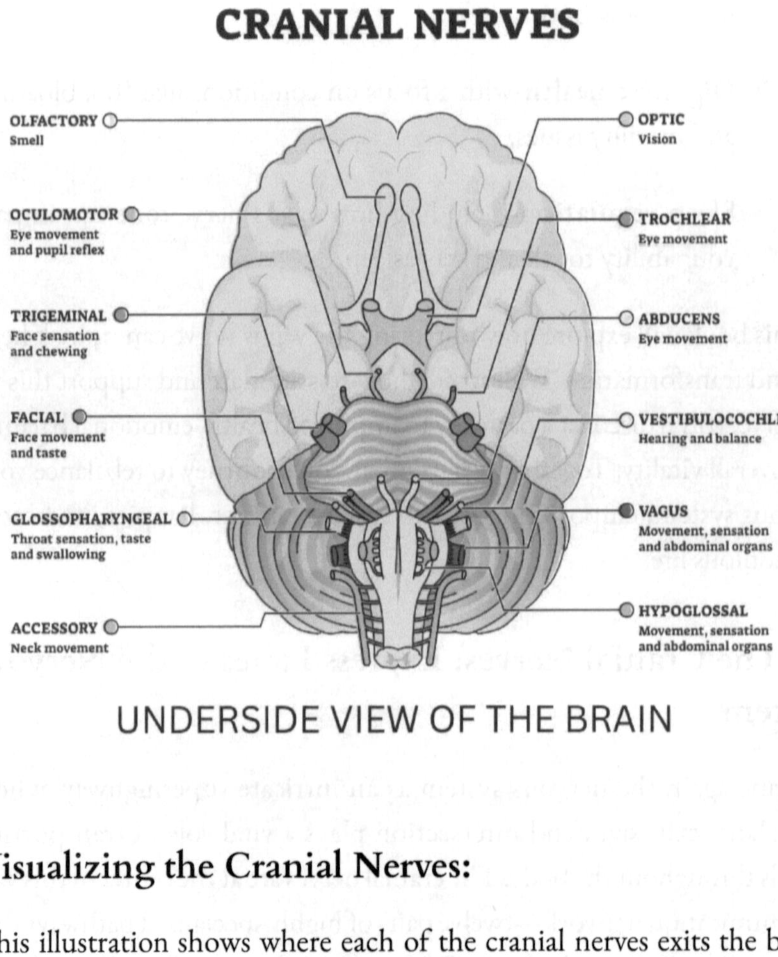

Visualizing the Cranial Nerves:

This illustration shows where each of the cranial nerves exits the brain, viewed from the underside. By appreciating the complexity and strategic positioning of these nerves, we gain a deeper understanding of how our nervous system manages a wide range of vital functions—from facial expressions and sensory perception to heart rate and digestion.

To truly grasp how these nerves operate, it helps to visualize their pathways as if you're looking at a detailed city map. Each cranial nerve functions like an express lane, with clearly marked destinations-some controlling motor function, others transmitting sensory input, and several coordinating automatic internal processes. These fast, specialized routes keep the body running smoothly and in balance.

In the following section, you'll find a clear overview of each cranial nerve, along with details that highlight their unique roles. This foundational knowledge will help you better understand how closely your brain is connected to the rest of your body—and how essential these pathways are for health and harmony.

1. **Olfactory Nerve (I)**–The first cranial nerve is solely dedicated to the sense of smell. Imagine this as the sensory system that detects different aromas, from fresh flowers to burning toast, sending signals directly to the brain's olfactory bulb for processing.

2. **Optic Nerve (II)**–Responsible for vision, this nerve carries information from the eyes to the brain, similar to a high-speed fiber-optic cable transmitting real-time video data.

3. **Oculomotor Nerve (III)**–This nerve controls most of the eye's muscles and adjusts pupil size, ensuring precise and coordinated movements.

4. **Trochlear Nerve (IV)**–A specialist in eye movement, the trochlear nerve controls a single muscle that allows the eye to move downward and inward.

5. **Trigeminal Nerve (V)**–The largest cranial nerve is responsible for facial sensations and movements such as biting and chewing. It acts like a highly tuned sensory and motor highway connecting the face to the brain.

6. **Abducens Nerve (VI)**–This nerve controls a muscle that moves the eye outward, playing a crucial role in horizontal eye movements.

7. **Facial Nerve (VII)**–Essential for facial expressions, this nerve allows us to smile, frown, and convey emotions. It also plays a role in taste perception from the front two-thirds of the tongue.

8. **Vestibulocochlear Nerve (VIII)**–This dual-purpose nerve is vital for hearing and balance. It helps transmit sound waves from the inner ear to the brain and maintains equilibrium, preventing dizziness and unsteadiness.

9. **Glossopharyngeal Nerve (IX)**–This nerve assists with swallowing, salivation, and taste from the back one-third of the tongue. It also has a role in monitoring blood pressure and oxygen levels in the bloodstream.

10. **Vagus Nerve (X)**–The tenth cranial nerve, often called the "wandering nerve," extends far beyond the head and neck, influencing vital organs in the chest and abdomen. As I mentioned earlier, this nerve plays a crucial role in regulating autonomic functions, such as heart rate, digestion, and immune response. It also contributes to emotional regulation, acting as a calming force that helps the body recover from stress and maintain homeostasis.

11. **Accessory Nerve (XI)**-This nerve controls the muscles in the neck and shoulders, facilitating head and shoulder movements.

12. **Hypoglossal Nerve (XII)**–Responsible for tongue movements, the hypoglossal nerve enables speech, swallowing, and other motor functions involving the tongue.

The Significance of the Vagus Nerve:

Among the twelve cranial nerves, the vagus nerve (cranial nerve X) is particularly noteworthy due to its extensive reach and diverse responsibilities. It functions like a major highway that connects multiple city centers, ensuring that different systems work in harmony. Due to its role in the autonomic nervous system, the vagus nerve is also closely linked to stress responses and relaxation, making it a key player in overall health and well-being.

1.5 The Critical Role of the Gut-Brain Axis

In the intricate web of human biology, the gut-brain axis exemplifies the body's interconnectedness. This bidirectional communication system links the gastrointestinal tract (gut) with the central nervous system (brain). It's not a one-way street but a constant dialogue in which the gut informs the brain about digestion, immunity, and emotional states-and the brain, in turn, influences gut function, mood, and behavior. This axis plays a crucial role in regulating digestion, immune health, and emotional well-being.

What is the Gut-Brain Axis?

The gut-brain axis is a dynamic network of neural, chemical, and immune pathways:

- **Neural Communication:** The vagus nerve is the primary highway of this system, transmitting signals between the brain and the gut. It detects sensations like fullness, discomfort, or inflammation and relays this information to the brain, which, in turn, sends commands that influence digestive function and gut motility.

- **Chemical Messengers:** Neurotransmitters and hormones play a key role in this relationship. Remarkably, the gut produces many of the same neurotransmitters found in the brain, such as serotonin, dopamine, and GABA-all of which regulate mood, sleep, and behavior.

- **Immune Pathways:** About 70% of the immune system resides in the gut. Immune cells in the intestinal lining send messages to the brain, influencing inflammatory responses, immunity, and even mood.

- **Digestive and Microbial Functions:** The gut microbiome-a diverse ecosystem of trillions of bacteria, viruses, and fungi-produces essential nutrients, breaks down complex carbohydrates, and generates short-chain fatty acids that feed gut cells and modulate inflammation.

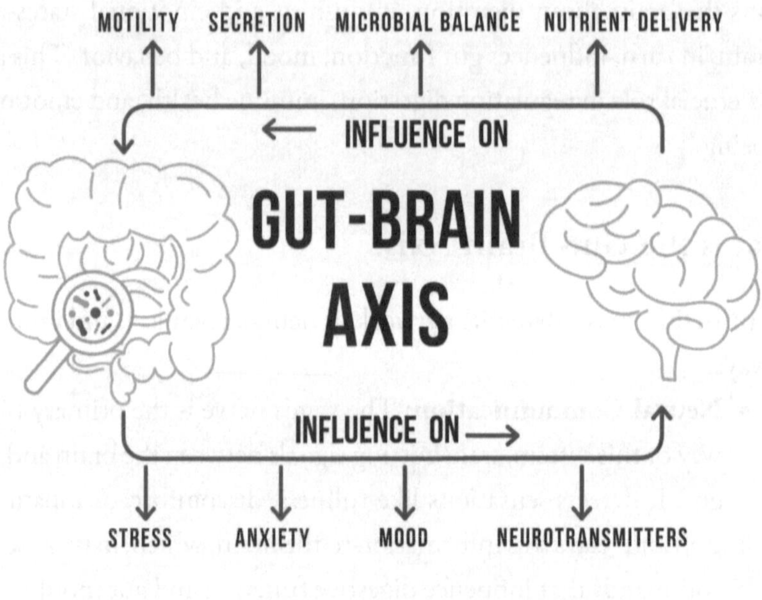

Example: Approximately 90% of the body's serotonin-a key mood regulator-is produced in the gut. When gut bacteria are out of balance, serotonin production can be disrupted, contributing to anxiety or depression.

The Stress-Gut Feedback Loop

At the heart of the gut-brain axis is the stress feedback loop, which demonstrates how emotions influence digestion and vice versa.

- **Gut to Brain:** The vagus nerve detects gut imbalances, such as inflammation, microbial shifts, or bloating, and sends distress signals to the brain, which can lead to mood changes or fatigue.

- **Brain to Gut:** Stress activates the sympathetic nervous system, triggering the release of cortisol and adrenaline, which can reduce digestive secretions, alter gut motility, and lead to symptoms such as nausea, cramping, or diarrhea.

Example: After a stressful event, your brain may signal a decrease in blood flow to the digestive tract. This "emergency override" can temporarily halt digestion, which is why anxiety often causes stomach upset.

Dysbiosis: When Balance Is Lost

Dysbiosis is a disruption in the healthy balance of the gut microbiome. It can stem from a poor diet, stress, the use of antibiotics, a lack of sleep, and exposure to environmental toxins.

- **Digestive Symptoms:** Bloating, gas, constipation, diarrhea, indigestion, food intolerances

- **Increased Gut Permeability:** Also known as "leaky gut," this allows toxins and pathogens to enter the bloodstream, triggering systemic inflammation and immune dysfunction

- **Beyond the Gut:** Fatigue, brain fog, skin issues, joint pain, anxiety, depression, and weight imbalances

Example: Research shows that people with anxiety and depression often have less microbial diversity and higher levels of inflammatory bacteria in their gut.

The Gut-Brain Axis and Mental Health

The enteric nervous system (ENS), often referred to as the "second-brain," governs digestion independently but is profoundly influenced by signals from the vagus nerve and microbial activity. Many mental health conditions are linked to disruptions in this axis:

- **Serotonin:** Regulates mood, sleep, and appetite; 90% made in the gut
- **Dopamine:** Influences motivation and reward; shaped by gut bacteria
- **GABA:** Calms the nervous system; supported by healthy microbial function

Example: Chronic stress can damage the gut lining and reduce serotonin and GABA levels, contributing to low mood, anxiety, or insomnia.

Nurturing the Gut-Brain Axis: Evidence-Based Strategies

Understanding the gut-brain connection allows us to take tangible steps to support both physical and emotional health. Here are evidence-based ways to nurture this vital relationship:

Prioritize a Balanced Diet with Prebiotics and Probiotics: Focus on a diverse, whole-food diet rich in fiber, fruits, vegetables, and fermented foods like yogurt, kefir, and sauerkraut. Include prebiotic fibers from foods such as bananas, garlic, and onions to nourish beneficial gut bacteria and promote microbiome diversity. A healthy diet fuels your microbiome, supporting digestion and emotional balance.

Incorporate Stress Management Practices: Engage in relaxation techniques such as deep breathing, meditation, or yoga to activate the vagus nerve and support the function of the parasympathetic nervous system. Managing stress helps regulate your nervous system and improves gut health.

Engage in Regular Exercise: Physical activity enhances gut microbiome diversity and reduces stress, anxiety, and depression. Movement helps modulate neurotransmitter levels and strengthens gut-brain communication.

Aim for Adequate Sleep: Strive for 7–9 hours of restorative sleep to maintain gut-brain communication and support hormonal balance. A good night's sleep restores bodily systems and promotes emotional resilience.

Conclusion: Harmonizing the Gut-Brain Connection

The gut-brain axis highlights the profound interconnection between physical and mental health. Maintaining a balanced gut microbiome and supporting clear communication between the gut and brain can enhance digestion, boost immune function, and improve emotional well-being. This holistic approach fosters vitality by embracing the powerful link between the gut, brain, and nervous system.

In the next section, we'll take a closer look at neurotransmitters—what they are, how they function, and how they influence nearly every aspect of your health.

1.6 More About Neurotransmitters

In the intricate dance of human biology, neurotransmitters serve as the messengers of the nervous system. They are chemical messengers that your body cannot live without. They ensure seamless communication between nerve cells (neurons), muscle cells, or glands. They are classified based on their chemical structure or their function. Without going into further detail and running the risk of confusing you, let's talk about them according to their function: inhibitory, excitatory, and modulating communication. Sometimes, a neurotransmitter can have both inhibitory and excitatory functions, depending on its location in the body. For now, imagine them as couriers in a bustling city, delivering messages that dictate everything from your mood and thoughts to your heartbeat and muscle movements. Without these chemical messengers, the nervous system would be like a vast metropolis without any means of transportation—no cars, trains, buses, or subways—making coordination and daily functions impossible.

But how exactly do neurotransmitters work? Neurotransmitters are chemical messengers produced by neurons (nerve cells) that transmit signals across synapses, the tiny gaps between nerve cells. A synapse is a bridge that allows information to pass from one neuron to another. Neurotransmitters carry messages across this bridge to another neuron, and this bridging process can be repeated until the signal reaches its destination, a muscle cell or a gland, allowing neurons to communicate effectively throughout our bodies.

Example: Imagine sending a text message. The phone (neuron) creates the message (neurotransmitter), sends it through the network (synapse), and another phone (neuron) receives it, which interprets and responds to the message. Like this communication flow, neurotransmitters send signals influencing thoughts, feelings, and bodily functions.

The Role of Neurotransmitters in the Autonomic Nervous System (ANS)

We've already discussed neurotransmitters in general, but it is essential to understand how these neurotransmitters function within the autonomic nervous system (ANS). Remember, this is the part of the nervous system that controls involuntary bodily functions, and neurotransmitters are the key players that regulate both the sympathetic and parasympathetic divisions.

Sympathetic Nervous System (SNS): The Body's Accelerator

The SNS is your body's "fight or flight" system. It prepares you to react to stress or danger, enhancing your alertness and physical readiness.

•Key Neurotransmitters:

Norepinephrine and epinephrine (adrenaline) are the primary excitatory neurotransmitters that activate the body's stress response. They increase heart rate, raise blood pressure, and redirect blood flow to muscles, preparing the body for quick action.

□ Think of norepinephrine as the loud alarm clock that jolts you out of sleep, instantly making you alert and ready to face the day.

□ Epinephrine is like stepping on the gas pedal of a race car, giving you the burst of energy needed to escape danger or face a challenge head-on.

Example: If you encounter a growling dog, your sympathetic nervous system releases norepinephrine and epinephrine, which increases your heart rate and pumps more blood to your muscles, preparing you to either run away or defend yourself.

Parasympathetic Nervous System (PNS): The Body's Brake

The PNS is the "rest and digest" system. It helps the body relax and recover once the perceived threat has passed. It slows the heart rate, stimulates digestion, and promotes a state of calmness.

•Key Neurotransmitter:

Acetylcholine is the primary neurotransmitter in the parasympathetic system. It is inhibitory and calming, slowing down the heart rate.

o Imagine acetylcholine as a soothing lullaby, helping your body relax after a stressful event, like gently pressing the brake pedal to slow down a speeding car.

o Outside of the vagus nerve's impact on the heart in the parasympathetic system, acetylcholine can be an excitatory neurotransmitter in the autonomic nervous system, impacting the parasympathetic and sympathetic nervous systems.

Example: After escaping the growling dog and reaching a safe place, acetylcholine is released, helping your heart rate return to normal and allowing you to catch your breath and calm down.

The Adrenal Glands: Powerhouse of Neurotransmitter Production

The adrenal glands on top of your kidneys are vital in producing neurotransmitters, especially during the body's stress response.

•Adrenal Medulla: This inner part of the adrenal gland releases epinephrine and norepinephrine into the bloodstream when you face a threat or stressful situation.

o It acts like a turbo boost in a video game, giving your body a surge of energy to react swiftly to danger.

o This rapid release amplifies the "fight or flight" response, increasing alertness, heart rate, and blood flow to muscles, preparing you to confront the danger or escape.

Example: If you're startled by a loud noise, your adrenal medulla releases a burst of epinephrine and norepinephrine, causing your heart to race and your muscles to tense, preparing you to react quickly.

Other Crucial Neurotransmitters and Their Functions

Dopamine: The Motivation and Reward Messenger

•Dopamine is often called the "feel-good" neurotransmitter because of its role in pleasure and reward. It also regulates movement, attention, and learning.

•Imagine dopamine as the applause you receive after achieving something significant, motivating you to continue pursuing your goals.

•In the ANS, dopamine also influences blood flow and the release of other neurotransmitters.

•It can be excitatory or inhibitory depending upon the type of receptor it binds to.

Example: When you eat your favorite dessert or achieve a long-sought goal, dopamine is released, giving you a sense of pleasure and satisfaction.

Serotonin: The Mood Stabilizer

•Serotonin helps regulate mood, sleep, appetite, and digestion. It promotes feelings of well-being and happiness.

•Think of serotonin as the sunlight on a beautiful morning, lifting your mood and helping you feel calm and content.

•Serotonin can be excitatory or inhibitory depending on the receptor it binds to.

Example: After a good workout, serotonin levels increase, leaving you feeling relaxed and happy, often called the "post-exercise high."

GABA (Gamma-Aminobutyric Acid): The Calming Agent

•GABA is an inhibitory neurotransmitter that slows down brain activity, helping you relax and reducing anxiety.

•Imagine GABA as a soothing cup of herbal tea that enables you to unwind and sleep peacefully.

Example: Before bedtime, GABA levels rise, quieting the mind and facilitating a transition into restful sleep.

The Balance of Excitatory and Inhibitory Neurotransmitters

•Excitatory Neurotransmitters (like epinephrine and norepinephrine) stimulate the nervous system, increasing alertness and energy.

•Inhibitory Neurotransmitters (like GABA) calm the nervous system, reducing anxiety and promoting relaxation.

This delicate balance between excitatory and inhibitory signals is crucial for maintaining homeostasis, the body's state of internal stability. An imbalance can lead to mental health issues, sleep disturbances, or chronic stress.

Example: In anxiety disorders or ADHD, an imbalance between excitatory and inhibitory neurotransmitters can cause overstimulation, leading to restlessness and nervousness.

Review of Neurotransmitters

Let's review the neurotransmitters and some of their variety of functions.

Norepinephrine- increases alertness and wakefulness and stimulates various processes in the body.

Epinephrine stimulates the fight-or-flight response, increasing heart rate, breathing, blood pressure, and glucose production.

Acetylcholine is essential for muscle function, regulates your sleep cycle, and is excitatory in all cases except for the heart, which is inhibitory.

Dopamine- is responsible for reward, motivation, and muscle movement and is both inhibitory and excitatory.

Serotonin regulates mood, sleep, pain, body temperature, and appetite and exhibits both inhibitory and excitatory effects.

GABA is the primary inhibitory neurotransmitter responsible for calming and reducing anxiety.

The Symphony of Neurotransmitters

Balance is key.

When neurotransmitters are functioning properly, the body remains in harmony. Too much or too little of any one neurotransmitter can result in symptoms such as:

- Mood swings
- Insomnia or fatigue
- Poor concentration
- Nervous system overstimulation or suppression and more

Example: Chronic stress often leads to reduced serotonin and GABA, while increasing norepinephrine. This imbalance may result in anxiety, digestive upset, or insomnia.

Maintaining neurotransmitter health involves:

- Nutritional support (e.g., amino acids, B vitamins, magnesium)
- Gut health optimization
- Adequate sleep and exercise
- Mind-body practices that improve vagal tone and reduce stress

Understanding the roles of neurotransmitters offers a glimpse into the elegant dance of signals that govern our daily lives. These chemical messengers enable us to adapt, thrive, and find balance amidst life's challenges. By appreciating their functions, we gain deeper insight into the forces within us that shape our health and well-being.

As we continue our journey, we will explore how nurturing the vagus nerve—the master regulator of the autonomic nervous system (ANS)—can harmonize this intricate superhighway system, leading to profound shifts in physical and emotional well-being.

Conclusion: A New Lens on Healing

The nervous system is more than a biological system—it is your body's communication hub, deeply intertwined with every function, sensation, and emotion you experience. By understanding how the central and peripheral nervous systems interact, and how the vagus nerve influences this interaction, you gain clarity into why certain symptoms appear and how healing unfolds. Whether you're dealing with digestive issues, anxiety, pain, or fatigue, reconnecting with your nervous system gives you the power to make lasting, meaningful changes in your health.

Now that you understand the broader nervous system landscape, it's time to explore the main character in this story: the vagus nerve. In Chapter 2, we'll dive deep into its structure, pathways, and function. You'll learn why it's called the "wandering nerve," how it interfaces with vital organs, and why it's considered the master regulator of your internal balance. Let's continue our journey by uncovering the incredible design and influence of this essential nerve.

Chapter 2: The Amazing Vagus Nerve Unveiled

Once again, imagine you are on a long, winding road trip, weaving through breathtaking landscapes of mountains and valleys. Each twist and turn takes you closer to your destination, offering new surprises and challenges. This journey mirrors the vagus nerve, also known as the wandering or roaming nerve, which stretches from the brainstem to the abdomen. The vagus nerve influences nearly every vital organ, forming an essential communication highway connecting bustling cities and serene countryside throughout the body. The vagus nerve's journey is not just about distance; it's about the profound connections it forms throughout the body that influence your physical and mental/emotional landscape.

2.1 The Journey Begins:

The word "vagus" originates from the Latin term for "wandering," a fitting description for a nerve that travels more extensively than any other cranial nerve. In terms of sheer reach, the vagus nerves span approximately 18-24 inches within the body, depending upon your height and anatomy. This impressive length allows it to serve as a primary conduit for communication between the brain and the body's organs, like a major interstate that ensures smooth traffic flow across states. Its fibers are a mix of sensory and motor pathways, allowing it to send and receive information and ensuring that your body maintains balance and harmony.

2.2 The Structure of the Vagus Nerve

Below is a picture of the brain and the vagus nerve, along with its connected organs, to give you an idea of the magnitude, complexity, and reach.

The Brain and Vagus Nerves

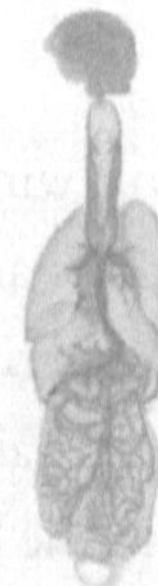

Think of it as if your body as a city, with the vagus nerve functioning as a complex highway system ensuring smooth traffic flow. Here are the parts of the vagus nerve system.

Vagus Nerve = A Major Interstate Superhighway

The vagus nerve is like a massive interstate highway that extends from the brain (the central hub) down through the neck, chest, and abdomen. It carries important messages between the brain and various organs, like an interstate connecting major cities, rest stops, and smaller roads, ultimately leading to specific destinations, structures, and organs.

Vagal Nerve Plexuses = Highway Interchanges

Along the way, the vagus nerve branches out and forms plexuses, such as those in the esophagus, heart, and intestines. These plexuses are simply an interconnected mass of nerve fibers acting as large highway interchanges where nerve signals merge, reorganize, and continue to their destinations, ensuring smooth communication between different organ systems.

Vagal Ganglia = Rest Stops & Control Centers

The vagus nerve has ganglia, such as the superior and inferior vagal ganglia, which act as rest stops and control centers where nerve signals pause, process information, and sometimes reroute. These ganglia help regulate sensory information from the body and fine-tune autonomic functions, such as heart rate, digestion, and inflammation control.

In short, the vagus nerve is your body's superhighway of communication. Its plexuses are the interchanges, and its ganglia are the rest stops and control centers, ensuring smooth traffic flow for vital body functions.

Dorsal and Ventral Branches

Return to the image in your mind of your body as a vast metropolitan area with the vagus nerve acting as a sophisticated system of highways, each lane bustling with signals like cars on a busy road. From its origin on the brainstem, each vagus nerve (right and left) splits into two primary branches, each serving distinct roles and destinations. These two highways branch off and extend their influence across the body, playing crucial roles in maintaining balance and function.

- Dorsal branch (back of the body pathway R and L):
    - This branch primarily connects to organs below the diaphragm (the muscle that divides our chest from our abdomen and is the primary muscle that makes breathing possible), including the digestive system. This branch is like a crucial service route for delivery trucks, ensuring that the organs (businesses) it reaches receive what they need to operate smoothly, facilitating digestion, nutrient absorption, and other essential processes.
    - It is crucial in the "freeze" response- a physiological pause button. When the body perceives an overwhelming threat, the "freeze" response, a paralyzing reaction, kicks in, slowing the heart rate and conserving energy. It's like hitting the brakes and stopping in heavy traffic to prevent an accident. This response is part of the body's survival mechanism, allowing it to remain still, quiet, and unmoving when faced with a threat or danger.

- Ventral branch (front of the body pathway R and L):
    - This branch connects to organs above the diaphragm, including the heart and lungs. This highway fosters a state of calm and connection. When you're relaxed, this branch helps maintain a steady heartbeat and smooth breathing, like cruising along a serene country road with the windows down.
    - It facilitates the "rest and digest" functions, allowing your body to recover and rejuvenate. This branch is crucial for emotional regulation and social interaction, contributing to feelings of safety and overall well-being. The ventral branch supports behaviors associated with connection and communication, enabling you to engage with others and manage stress effectively.

Understanding these pathways and their functions invites you to consider how deeply interconnected your body truly is. The dorsal branches roles in the "freeze" response and the ventral branches contribution to relaxation highlight the vagus nerve's versatility within your body's infrastructure. It's like having a built-in navigation system that adjusts your route based on current conditions, ensuring you arrive at your destination safely and efficiently. These pathways help modulate your physiological responses, allowing you to adapt to different situations with resilience and poise. The interplay between the dorsal and ventral branches illustrates the complexity of your body's internal network, where each component works in harmony to maintain balance and promote health.

Considering the vagus nerve's extensive reach, consider how its pathways might influence your daily life. Perhaps you've experienced moments of anxiety when your heart races or times of calm when deep breaths bring a sense of peace. These sensations reflect the vagus nerve's activity, reminding you of its presence and power. It's a reminder that your body possesses the innate ability to regulate itself, which can be nurtured and enhanced through understanding and practice. The vagus nerve's branching structure offers a window into the intricate web of connections that sustain your health, inviting you to appreciate the elegance of its design and the potential for healing it holds.

Through your further exploration, you'll gain insight into how the vagus nerve supports your body's ability to respond to life's challenges. Whether the dorsal branch's role is in survival or the ventral branch's influence on connection, each pathway contributes to a tapestry of responses that shape your experience. These branches are not just highways of communication; they are conduits of resilience and well-being, guiding you through life's twists and turns. As you continue reading, let these insights inspire your curiosity and empower you. I hope you will be encouraged to explore the potential of the vagus nerve to transform your health and enrich your life.

2.3 Key Branches and Their Functions

Imagine standing on a bustling train platform for a moment, where each train represents a signal traveling through the vagus nerve, a vital link between the brain and your body. Remember that the vagus nerve is often called the "wandering nerve" because it embarks on a fascinating and essential journey, beginning at the brainstem and extending through various body regions. As these trains traverse their paths, they perform critical functions, carrying messages to and from the brain, ensuring harmony and balance within your body. The vagus nerve is like a grand conductor, orchestrating a symphony of bodily functions that maintain your health and well-being.

The structures involved in this intricate pathway are as diverse as the stations on a train route. From the medulla (part of the brainstem that connects your brain to your spinal cord), the vagus nerve descends out of the skull and through the neck, nestled between the carotid artery and the internal jugular vein (the major vessels in your neck- the carotid is where you can feel your pulse), much like a commuter train weaving through a bustling cityscape. As its journey continues, the vagus nerve branches into various pathways, each with a distinct destination and purpose.

These branches are essential for regulating critical functions such as heart rate, digestion, and respiratory rate, like a network of trains ensuring the smooth operation of a vast transportation system. Remember, the nerves that branch off the vagus nerve, like major roads (six lanes), intersect with medium-sized roads (four lanes) and more minor roads, two-lane streets, leading to vital destinations, such as neighborhoods or businesses. We have major highway interchanges, and rest stops along the way. We will start from the head and work our way down. This drawing will help you to visualize these branches. I want you to know that the information that follows may seem complicated, but it becomes necessary for you to learn the anatomy and physiology associated with your health and well-being. You will start to see how important it is to take actions to restore function and balance to your body, instead of suffering with numerous symptoms and conditions only to watch your health get worse.

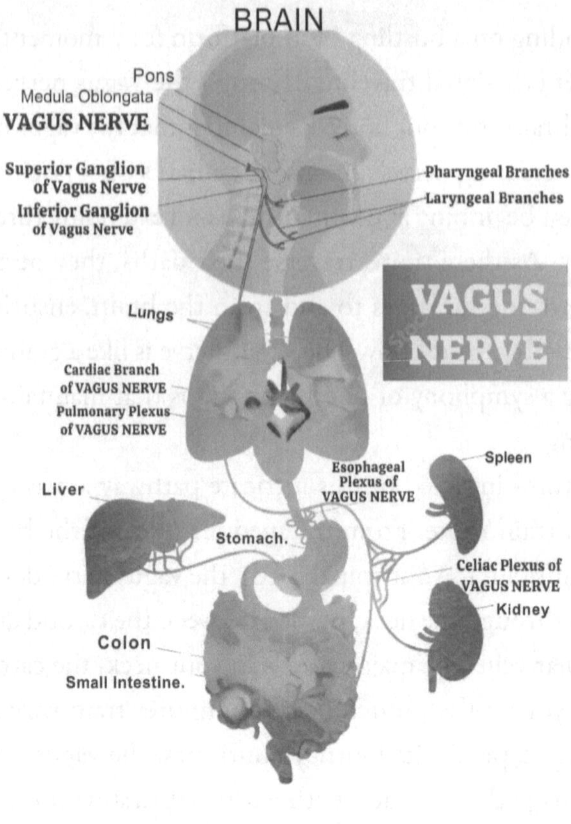

HEAD AND NECK BRANCHES

As we explore the vagus nerve's journey through the head and throat, we encounter fascinating branches and structures, each playing a unique role in maintaining balance and function. The auricular branch, also known as Arnold's nerve, is an intriguing component that provides sensory (touch) innervation to the skin of the ear canal, tragus (the part of the ear you push on to plug your ear), and auricle (or the pinna, the outer part of your ear). Picture it as a finely tuned sensor that detects subtle changes, sending signals back to the brain about the state of these areas. Interestingly, this nerve can also trigger a phenomenon known as the Ear-Cough or Arnold Reflex, where stimulation of the ear canal can elicit a cough. This curious reflex highlights the interconnectedness of our body's systems, reminding us that seemingly isolated areas can influence distant parts of the body.

Moving to the throat, the vagus nerve's pharyngeal (throat) branches step into the spotlight. These branches are responsible for innervating the muscles of the pharynx and palate (the roof of your mouth), excluding one muscle. Imagine the pharynx as a bustling highway interchange, where signals direct traffic to ensure smooth swallowing and proper speech. The coordination of these muscles is crucial for everyday activities, such as eating and speaking, allowing us to communicate and nourish ourselves with ease. When these branches function optimally, they facilitate seamless transitions between breathing, speaking, and swallowing, thereby maintaining the harmony of the intricate operations of our throats.

The superior laryngeal (larynx=voicebox where vocal cords are located) nerve, another significant branch of the vagus nerve, divides into internal and external branches, each with a distinct function. The internal branch supplies the mucous membrane of the larynx, providing sensory feedback that informs the brain about the state of the larynx. Meanwhile, the external branch innervates the cricothyroid muscle, a key player in voice modulation. This muscle adjusts the tension of the vocal cords, enabling us to produce a range of pitches and tones. Whether singing your favorite song or engaging in a heartfelt conversation, the superior laryngeal nerve ensures that your voice is expressive and resonant.

Within the complex web of the vagus nerve, the superior and inferior ganglia serve as critical junctions that help regulate breathing, speech, and sweating. Imagine these ganglia as communication hubs, where signals are relayed to ensure the body's responses are appropriate and timely. By regulating these vital functions, the ganglia play a crucial role in maintaining our body's equilibrium, allowing us to adapt to environmental changes quickly. Whether taking a deep breath before a presentation or cooling down after a brisk walk, these structures ensure that your body remains responsive and balanced.

CHEST BRANCHES

The vagus nerve branches continue their intricate path through the neck and into the chest and abdomen, forming networks that influence vital organs, each maintaining crucial equilibrium of the body. In the chest, the vagus nerve forms the pulmonary and cardiac plexuses, which manage the intricate functions of the heart and lungs. These plexuses are like major transit hubs, coordinating the flow of signals that regulate heart rate, respiratory rate, and blood pressure. These branches deliver parasympathetic signals that help regulate the heart rate and maintain a steady, calm beat. When you feel your heart slow after a fright or relax during a moment of peace, it's the cardiac branches at work. They ensure that your heart adapts to your body's needs, whether sitting quietly or engaging in physical activity. By modulating the heart's pace, these branches help balance energy conservation and readiness for action, an essential aspect of cardiovascular health.

In the bustling landscape of the chest, the pulmonary branches of the vagus nerve play their part, weaving through the lungs like a network of communication lines. These branches regulate the delicate balance between inhalation (breathing in) and exhalation (breathing out), ensuring smooth and efficient breathing. They send signals that influence the contraction and relaxation of the bronchial muscles, facilitating the flow of air into and out of the lungs. When you take a deep breath to calm yourself or feel the rush of air during exercise, you're experiencing the subtle control of the pulmonary branches. Their role extends beyond mere mechanics; they also help to modulate inflammatory responses within the lungs, supporting respiratory health and protecting against potential irritants. They also target secretory glands in the lungs, which increases the production of serous fluid, a thin layer of fluid that lubricates the lung membranes. This fluid helps the membranes to slide over each other during breathing. These branches also carry sensory information about stretch and irritation in the lungs. This feedback helps regulate the tone of the bronchial muscles and the cough reflex.

The esophageal branches of the vagus nerve are another fascinating component in this complex network. They oversee the coordinated movement of food and liquid from the throat to the stomach, which is known as peristalsis. These branches regulate swallowing and send rhythmic motor signals to the smooth muscles of the esophagus, which propel swallowed contents down the esophagus, ensuring that each meal travels smoothly and efficiently. This complex process also stimulates motility in the distal stomach, which aids in gastric emptying, increases mucus secretion in the esophagus, and relaxes the lower esophageal sphincter. (The muscle that controls your esophagus's connection to your stomach). Imagine these branches as skilled navigators, guiding each bite along a well-charted path to digestion. They work tirelessly to prevent disruptions, such as acid reflux or swallowing difficulties, that can arise when the esophagus's function is compromised. Beyond their digestive duties, these branches also provide sensory feedback to the brain, informing it of the esophagus's status and adjusting responses as needed.

Essentially, the vagus nerve's pathways through the neck and chest form a sophisticated network supporting vital bodily functions. Whether it's the consistent beat of your heart, the steady rhythm of your breath, or the smooth passage of food, these branches ensure that your body's internal environment remains balanced and responsive. By understanding the roles of these branches, you gain insight into the delicate interplay that sustains your health and well-being, inviting you to appreciate the remarkable connectivity within your body.

ABDOMINAL BRANCHES

Consider the vagus nerve's journey, which now extends deep into the abdomen, playing a pivotal role in your digestive health and overall well-being. It is a crucial component of the parasympathetic nervous system, orchestrating a wide range of autonomic functions that influence digestion, metabolism, and communication between organs. As the right and left vagus nerves continue their journey into the abdomen, they form the gastric, celiac, and hepatic branches, playing vital roles in regulating the gut-liver-brain axis, influencing everything from ensuring the efficient breakdown of food, the absorption of nutrients, and inflammation control much like the logistics of a well-organized supply chain.

Gastric Branches of the Vagus Nerve

Functions & Roles:

Stomach Innervation: The vagus nerve connects to the enteric nervous system (ENS), The enteric nervous system (ENS) is a complex network of neurons located within the walls of the gastrointestinal (GI) tract, it modulates the digestive process. It plays a crucial role in regulating digestion, absorption, and other gut functions.

Gastric Acid Secretion: It stimulates parietal cells, also known as oxyntic cells, that are stomach lining cells that produce hydrochloric acid (HCl) and intrinsic factor, which is essential for vitamin B12 absorption. Hydrochloric acid (HCl), which aids in protein breakdown and nutrient absorption (iron, B12).

Motility Control: Regulates gastric emptying and peristalsis, ensuring food moves efficiently from the stomach to the intestines.

Hunger and Satiation Regulation: This system communicates with the hypothalamus via gut hormones, including ghrelin (a hormone produced in your stomach that stimulates appetite and increases food intake), cholecystokinin (CCK) (a hormone produced in your small intestine that stimulate your gall bladder and pancreas to contract), and GLP-1, to signal hunger and fullness. GLP-1 has become well known as an injectable to assist people in losing weight.

Mucosal Protection & Healing: Helps maintain gastric mucosal integrity, reducing the risk of ulcers and gastritis. Mucosa refers to the moist, inner lining of various body cavities and organs, such as the mouth, nose, lungs, and stomach. It is a protective layer that secretes mucus, a thick and slippery substance, to lubricate and shield these surfaces from irritation and infection.

Imbalance & Dysfunction

When the vagal tone is low, or the gastric branch is dysfunctional, symptoms can manifest as:

Gastroparesis (Delayed Gastric Emptying): Slow stomach emptying causes bloating, nausea, and a sudden feeling of fullness.

Hypochlorhydria (Low Stomach Acid) – Impaired acid secretion can cause malabsorption of nutrients (iron, B12, zinc) and increased risk of infections (H. pylori, SIBO). SIBO stands for Small Intestine Baceterial Overwgrowth

Excess Acid Secretion & GERD – Imbalance can lead to acid reflux, damaging the esophageal lining.

MMC (Migrating Motor Complex) Disruption leads to bacterial overgrowth (SIBO) and impaired digestive clearance.

Increased Gut Inflammation can contribute to gastritis, ulcers, or autoimmune responses, such as celiac disease and Crohn's disease.

Celiac Branches of the Vagus Nerve

Functions & Roles:

Autonomic Control of the Intestines: This is part of the celiac plexus is a network of nerves located in the upper abdomen, behind the pancreas and near the aorta, that connects the pancreas, gallbladder, intestines, liver, and stomach to the brain and spinal cord, sending signals from these organs, which regulates them.

Intestinal Motility & Peristalsis: Ensures rhythmic contractions of the intestines to move food and prevent stagnation.

Gut-Immune Communication: Supports immune tolerance and controls inflammatory responses in the gut.

Microbiome Regulation: Influences the balance of gut bacteria, preventing dysbiosis and overgrowth of harmful microbes.

Pancreatic Function: It stimulates the pancreas to release digestive enzymes to breakdown food into nutrients and secrete insulin for blood sugar control.

Imbalance & Dysfunction

Dysfunction in the celiac branches can result in:

Irritable Bowel Syndrome (IBS) – Irregular motility leads to diarrhea, constipation, and bloating.

Small Intestinal Bacterial Overgrowth (SIBO) – Impaired motility allows bacteria to accumulate in the small intestine, causing bloating, gas, and malabsorption.

Leaky Gut (Increased Intestinal Permeability) – Weak vagal signaling disrupts gut lining integrity, contributing to autoimmune conditions.

Pancreatic Insufficiency – Reduced enzyme secretion impairs digestion, leading to nutrient deficiencies.

Hepatic Branches of the Vagus Nerve

Functions & Roles:

Liver-Brain Communication: The vagus nerve signals between the liver and hypothalamus (brain) and regulates glucose balance, metabolism, and immune responses.

Bile Secretion & Gallbladder Function: Controls bile release from the gallbladder to aid in the digestion of fats and fat-soluble vitamins (A, D, E, K).

Glucose and Lipid Metabolism: Modulate insulin sensitivity, affecting fat storage, blood sugar levels, and cholesterol balance.

Liver Detoxification Supports Phase I and II detox pathways, helping the body clear toxins, hormones, and metabolic waste.

Inflammation Control: Influences cytokine signaling to regulate systemic inflammation and immune function. Cytokines are small proteins secreted by cells that act as chemical messengers to communicate with and regulate other cells

Imbalance & Dysfunction

Dysfunction in the hepatic branch can result in:

Non-Alcoholic Fatty Liver Disease (NAFLD)– Poor vagal signaling impairs lipid metabolism, leading to fat accumulation in the liver.

Gallbladder Stasis and gallstones: Weak vagal activity can reduce bile flow, leading to bile stagnation and gallstone formation.

Blood Sugar Dysregulation & Insulin Resistance – Impaired vagal tone contributes to metabolic disorders like Type 2 diabetes.

Increased Systemic Inflammation can exacerbate autoimmune conditions, joint pain, and neuroinflammation.

Reduced Detoxification Efficiency – This reduction leads to hormone imbalances, skin issues, and a sluggish metabolism.

Key Takeaways & Clinical Relevance

1. The vagus nerve plays a central role in regulating digestion, metabolism, immunity, and inflammation through its gastric, celiac, and hepatic branches.
2. Dysfunction in these branches contributes to gut disorders (SIBO, GERD, IBS), metabolic disease (NAFLD, diabetes), and systemic inflammation.
3. Vagal Toning Techniques can enhance vagus nerve function, supporting optimal digestion, detoxification, and gut-brain health.

Some Ways to Strengthen Vagal Function

Diaphragmatic Breathing – Stimulates vagus nerve activity and enhances gut motility.

Cold Exposure – Activates parasympathetic tone and reduces inflammation.

Gargling & Humming stimulate vagal activation through vocal cord engagement.

Mindful Eating – Slows down digestion, improving gastric and pancreatic enzyme secretion.

Probiotic-Rich Foods – Supports a healthy gut microbiome, reinforcing gut-vagus communication.

Acupuncture & Auricular Vagus Nerve Stimulation (VNS) – Directly stimulates vagal pathways for digestive and metabolic balance.

As you can see, these pathways are pivotal in regulating many functions beyond digestion and nutrient absorption, like a finely tuned engine converting fuel into energy. By maintaining the delicate balance between various bodily functions, the vagus nerve acts as a guardian of homeostasis, ensuring that no system operates in isolation. Take a moment to go back and review the picture of the intricate branches of the vagus nerve.

As you continue to navigate your understanding of the vagus nerve, bring back to your mind the picture of it as a sophisticated network of highways and roads, each playing a crucial role in maintaining traffic flow within your body. This metaphorical journey highlights the complexity and importance of the vagus nerve, reminding you of the intricate connections that sustain life. Through this exploration, you'll learn to appreciate the vagus nerve as a physical structure and a vital lifeline that weaves through every aspect of your well-being. As we delve deeper into its structure and function, you'll gain the tools and insights necessary to harness its potential for healing and transformation.

A Personal Exploration

Please take a moment to consider the following questions, reflecting on your recent experiences, to fully appreciate the transformative power of the vagus nerve.

Do you wonder about your vagus nerve function?

Have there been moments when stress seemed to derail your body's balance?

What physical sensations did you notice, and how did they influence your emotions?

Taking a moment to jot down these reflections can provide valuable insights into how your vagus nerve might affect your daily life. By connecting your personal observations to the concepts discussed, you can begin to uncover patterns and understand the significant role and impact this nerve plays in your health.

2.4 The Vagus Nerve's Dual Nature: Efferent and Afferent Pathways

As we continue to explore the vagus nerve, it becomes increasingly clear that this nerve is not a one-way street but a dynamic two-lane highway bustling with activity. The vagus nerve's dual nature consists of efferent (motor) and afferent (sensory) pathways, each playing a crucial role in maintaining the body's balance and function. Imagine these pathways as the nerves' communication lines, constantly sending and receiving signals to ensure your body operates smoothly. Now you can start to see what I've been explaining, interconnectes an works together.

Efferent (Motor) Pathways: The Nerve's Outgoing Signals

- Efferent pathways of the vagus nerve carry instructions from the brain to the organs, instructing them on how to function.
- These signals are essential in regulating involuntary actions like heartbeat, digestion, and respiration. When you take a deep breath to calm yourself, the vagus nerve's efferent pathways are at work, signaling the lungs to expand and the heart to slow down, promoting relaxation. This motor command enables your body to respond effectively to the demands of everyday life, ensuring that each organ plays its part in maintaining overall health.
- Interestingly, the Efferent Pathways play a vital role in vocalization and communication. Like we talked about earlier in the chapter, when you speak, hum, or sing, the vagus nerve sends signals to your vocal cords, coordinating their movement and modulating pitch, tone, and resonance. This intricate connection between the brain and the voice box highlights the nerve's multifaceted role

in internal and external communication. Beyond its impact on speech and sound production, the vagus nerve is deeply intertwined with emotional expression, helping to regulate vocal tone in response to mood and social interactions.

- Additionally, these motor pathways extend their influence beyond the voice, playing a key role in digestive function. The vagus nerve plays a crucial role in regulating the production of digestive enzymes, stomach acid secretion, and the rhythmic contractions of the gastrointestinal tract, peristalsis. Ensuring food moves efficiently from the esophagus to the stomach and through the intestines supports optimal nutrient absorption and waste elimination. This seamless coordination is essential for maintaining energy balance, gut health, and overall well-being.

Afferent (Sensory) Pathways: The Nerve's Incoming Signals

On the other hand, the afferent pathways of the vagus nerve are like the inbound messages, carrying sensory information from the body back to the brain.

- Make up 80% of vagus nerve total fibers, constantly monitoring the body's internal state.

- These pathways act as vigilant observers, constantly gathering data about the body's condition and reporting it to the brain. They provide feedback on various physiological parameters, such as heart rate, blood pressure, gut distension, chemical composition, and immune responses, allowing the brain to make informed decisions about maintaining homeostasis, the body's balance.

- This sensory information is critical for your brain to assess the body's needs and adjust its responses accordingly. When you feel the warmth of sitting by a fire wrapped in a cozy blanket or the fullness after a delicious dessert, the vagus nerve's afferent pathways communicate these sensations to your brain. This feedback loop is crucial for hunger regulation, enabling the brain to determine when to eat and stop eating.

- Influence emotional processing, linking gut sensations to mood ("gut feelings").

2.5 Review of the Vagus Nerve's Role and Structure

In the Autonomic Nervous System

The vagus nerve is the ultimate guardian of homeostasis, keeping the body's systems synchronized and responsive. This structural framework highlights the nerve's adaptive capacity, allowing us to efficiently navigate stress and relaxation states. Below is a summary of its role in the Autonomic Nervous System (ANS).

Sympathetic response ("fight or flight") – Prepares the body for danger by increasing heart rate and blood pressure.

Parasympathetic response ("rest and digest") is a standard baseline state of the parasympathetic nervous system. It includes the "freeze" response, an extreme, survival-oriented reaction to a perceived threat involving the parasympathetic nervous system, but in a different way, promoting relaxation, digestion, and healing.

Remember, the vagus nerve is the primary driver of the parasympathetic system, acting as a counterbalance to stress responses.

Vagus Nerve Structure

By promoting such a wide range of functions, the vagus nerve emerges as a central player in the body's two-way communication highway, carrying information between the brain and the body. These pathways ensure that the brain remains informed and responsive to changes in the body's environment. So, let's review what we have learned about the vagus nerve's structure. The right and left vagus nerves leave the medulla (part of the brainstem), and each of these branches splits into a dorsal (back) and ventral (front) nerve. Each major branch is further divided into smaller branches, which in turn branch into smaller branches to reach specific structures or organs. Each branch is a two-way street carrying both sensory and motor fibers to sense and respond to what is happening at that organ or structure. Also, remember that this communication network includes the Autonomic Nervous System functions, such as Fight or Flight, Rest and Digest, and the "Freeze" response. The vagus nerve's dual pathway creates a dialogue between the brain and the organs, fostering a harmonious balance that supports health and well-being. This intricate interplay of motor and sensory functions highlights the vagus nerve's versatility and stresses its importance in maintaining the body's equilibrium.

2.6 Special Sensory Functions

Beyond the extensive reach we have discussed, the vagus nerve has several specialized sensory functions associated with specialized sensory neurons (nerve cells).

- The vagus nerve contributes to taste perception by innervating the epiglottis (the flap at the back of the throat that prevents food and liquid from entering your lungs) and the back of the tongue. When you savor the flavors of a delicious meal, the vagus nerve is involved in transmitting taste signals to the brain, enhancing your culinary experience.

- It also plays a role in detecting chemical changes in the blood, helping regulate metabolic balance.

- Studies suggest vagal stimulation may enhance neuroplasticity, impacting memory and learning, which talk about more in an upcoming chapter.

This sensory connection highlights the nerve's role in physiological regulation and sensory perception, thereby bridging the gap between the body's internal functions and the external world.

2.7 Feedback and External Stimuli Impacting the Vagus Nerve

The vagus nerve is crucial in maintaining the delicate balance that keeps our bodies functioning optimally. This delicate balance is achieved through a series of continuously adjusting homeostatic feedback loops. A homeostatic feedback loop is a system that regulates body functions to maintain a stable internal environment. Imagine these loops as numerous ongoing conversations between your brain and your organs, where each part listens and responds to the other to maintain a state of balance. The vagus nerve acts as a mediator in these conversations, ensuring that any shifts from the norm are quickly addressed and corrected. For instance, if your heart rate spikes in response to an unexpected stressor, the vagus nerve sends signals to help return it to a resting state, thereby preserving overall well-being. This constant monitoring and adjusting are vital for health, allowing the body to adapt to daily changes and challenges. Homeostasis is a foundational characteristic of our bodies and lives; feedback loops are key to maintaining it.

External stimuli significantly influence the activity of the vagus nerve. Our modern lifestyle, filled with stress and fast-paced living, can easily disrupt the communication pathways within our nervous system. Stress profoundly impacts the vagus nerve, often reducing its tone and making it less effective at regulating bodily functions. When stress becomes chronic, it can lead to a cascade of effects, including elevated heart rates, shallow breathing, and impaired digestion, all of which can leave you feeling out of sorts. However, relaxation techniques, such as deep breathing and meditation, can counteract these effects by stimulating the vagus nerve, helping to restore balance and promote a sense of calm. These practices encourage the body to engage its natural healing mechanisms, lowering heart rates, improving respiratory efficiency, and enhancing nutrient absorption in the gut.

Understanding the feedback loop mechanism and the influence of external stimuli on the vagus nerve emphasizes the complexity of our bodies and the interconnectedness of our systems. By tuning into these signals and making mindful adjustments to our lifestyles, we can harness the power of the vagus nerve to support our health. This knowledge empowers us to make informed decisions about our well-being and highlights the potential for positive change through small, intentional actions. The vagus nerve reminds us of the body's innate capacity for balance and healing, encouraging us to nurture this vital connection for a healthier life.

Inflammation and Immune Regulation

Additionally, the vagus nerve plays a pivotal role in regulating inflammation and the immune response. It's like a vigilant police patrol, always looking for signs of trouble. When inflammation occurs as a response to injury or infection, the vagus nerve helps modulate this response, ensuring it doesn't become excessive or chronic, which could lead to further health issues. This regulation is part of the body's innate ability to protect itself while preventing damage from excessive or overreactive responses. By keeping inflammation in check, the vagus nerve supports healing processes. It maintains a robust immune system, ready to defend against pathogens while avoiding unnecessary harm to the body's tissues. Imagine your immune system as a vigilant highway patrol, looking out for potential lawbreakers or accidents, such as infections or injuries. The vagus nerve acts like a sophisticated communication network, sending signals that fine-tune the immune response, balancing aggression and caution.

So, when your body encounters a threat, the immune system springs into action, deploying white blood cells to the site of injury or infection.

These cells, the frontline soldiers of your body's defenses, work tirelessly to neutralize invaders and repair tissue. However, this process can sometimes lead to excessive inflammation, like a security team overreacting to a minor issue. The vagus nerve is activated here, releasing acetylcholine that controls the production of cytokines— the proteins that signal immune cells to increase their activity. By modulating cytokine production, the vagus nerve helps prevent the immune response from becoming too intense, reducing the risk of chronic inflammation and autoimmune disorders.

Moreover, the vagus nerve's engagement in the inflammatory reflex-a feedback loop that helps manage inflammation-illustrates its sophisticated role in immune regulation. This reflex involves sensing inflammation through afferent pathways and sending signals back through efferent pathways to dampen the immune response. It's like having a thermostat that adjusts the temperature based on the current climate, ensuring the environment remains neither too hot nor too cold. This mechanism is crucial for maintaining homeostasis, preventing the immune system from causing unnecessary damage to healthy tissues.

In addition to controlling inflammation, the vagus nerve also influences the production and release of other key immune components. For instance, it affects the activity of macrophages, the cells responsible for engulfing and digesting pathogens (pathogens are like a tiny germ, like a bacteria, virus, or fungus that can make you sick by causing harm or disease). By modulating the activity of these cells, the vagus nerve supports efficient pathogen clearance without excessive collateral damage, promoting healing and recovery. This regulation is critical in conditions characterized by chronic inflammation, where unchecked immune activity can lead to tissue damage and disease progression.

The vagus nerve's role in immune regulation highlights its importance in maintaining overall health. By preventing excessive inflammation and modulating the immune response, it helps protect the body from the harmful effects of chronic inflammation and autoimmunity. This intricate balance once again highlights the interconnectedness of our body's systems, where the nervous and immune systems collaborate to support health and resilience. Understanding this relationship empowers you to appreciate the multifaceted role of the vagus nerve in your well-being, inviting you to explore practices that nurture this vital connection.

Impact of Lifestyle Factors

Many factors can impact the vagus nerve, tone, and activation- its overall health. Here are just a few examples of lifestyle changes that anyone can make to help balance the vagus nerve. I will touch upon these topics, but I will expand upon these in much more detail as well as have additional information in my next book, "My Holistic Vagus Nerve Toolkit: A Naturopathic Doctor's Strategies to Promote & Restore Nervous System Balance for Digetive Health, Decreased Pain and Inflammation, Mental/Emotional Well-Being."

- Stress-reducing techniques-Chronic stress reduces vagal tone, impairing the body's ability to regulate heart rate, digestion, and sleep. To combat this, try interacting regularly with loved ones and friends and engaging in enjoyable activities.

- Deep breathing and meditation -Stimulate vagal activation, lower stress hormones, and enhance relaxation.

- Anti-inflammatory diet -An anti-inflammatory diet that avoids processed foods and refined carbohydrates, such as white bread and pastries, can help improve inflammation and vagal tone. Instead, eating a diet rich in fresh, organic foods, whenever possible, is essential. For example, a diet rich in anti-inflammatory foods like leafy greens, fatty fish, berries, and nuts can support the vagus nerve by reducing systemic inflammation and promoting healthy digestive function.

- Exercise-Regular physical activity is a natural stimulator of the vagus nerve, which boosts its tone and enhances overall resilience. Exercise encourages the release of endorphins, which positively affect mood and stress levels and reduce inflammation, further supporting the nerve's function.

These lifestyle changes can significantly enhance your body's ability to maintain homeostasis, fostering a healthier, more balanced state.

Techniques to Enhance Vagus Nerve Function

- Cold exposure (e.g., cold showers) – Stimulates the vagus nerve to improve stress resilience.
- Humming, chanting, or singing – Engages the nerve through vocal cord activation.
- Gargling – Stimulates the vagus nerve via throat muscles.

Conclusion: Unlocking the Power of the Vagus Nerve

As we conclude this chapter, we've unraveled the profound impact of the vagus nerve on our body's vital internal communication link between the brain and body, which is extensive and connects to many organs, regulating functions such as digestion, heart rate, breathing, inflammation, and immune function. Understanding its pathways and functions can help us tap into its transformative healing potential. Simple lifestyle modifications-stress reduction, mindful breathing, and dietary adjustments-can enhance vagal tone and promote resilience, balance, and overall well-being.

As we move forward, we'll explore how to recognize vagus nerve dysfunction and implement strategies for restoring balance in the body. But let's first talk about the vagus nerve's other functions. When they become disrupted, we can experience sleep disruption, anxiety, depression, and more. We'll also discuss how traumatic events and PTSD impact the vagus nerve's functioning.

Chapter 3: Rest, Digest, and Sleep—Your Body's Inner Conductor

Welcome to one of the most essential chapters in your journey of understanding the vagus nerve. This chapter explores the vagus nerve's foundational role in supporting three pillars of healing: rest, digestion, and sleep. These functions are not just bodily luxuries—they are biological necessities for survival, repair, and emotional resilience. The vagus nerve operates quietly beneath your awareness, orchestrating a delicate interplay between stress and restoration. By learning how this nerve contributes to your inner balance, you unlock powerful insights into your health and empower yourself with tools to live more harmoniously. Let's dive into how the vagus nerve helps you shift from chaos to calm, stress to serenity, and fatigue to deep, restorative rest.

3.1 Rest, Digest, and Sleep: The Vagus Nerve's Soothing Symphony

Imagine the vagus nerve as your body's personal symphony conductor, orchestrating a delicate balance between tension and tranquility. When you're overwhelmed with stress-your heart racing, breath shallow, muscles tense-the vagus nerve steps in like a skilled maestro, calming the cacophony and restoring harmony. It gently slows your heart, deepens your breath, and quiets your nervous system, much like a conductor soothing an over zealous orchestra into a peaceful melody.

This nerve is a core component of the parasympathetic nervous system-the "rest and digest" branch that counterbalances the "fight or flight" response. When activated, the vagus nerve sends calming signals throughout the body, lowering your heart rate, reducing blood pressure, and shifting you into a restorative state. It's like a soothing lullaby for your body, allowing you to unwind, heal, and rebuild from daily stressors. Without this calming influence, chronic stress can wear down the body, leading to emotional instability, inflammation, digestive issues, and sleep disturbances.

But the vagus nerve doesn't stop at relaxation-it plays a vital role indigestion as well. Picture your digestive system as a well-oiled engine. When you're calm and safe, the vagus nerve ensures this engine runs smoothly by triggering the release of digestive enzymes, stimulating bile flow, and promoting peristalsis-the rhythmic muscular contractions that move food through the gut. In this parasympathetic state, your body efficiently absorbs nutrients and eliminates waste, which is essential for energy, immune function, and metabolic balance. When the vagus nerve is underactive, digestion can falter, contributing to bloating, discomfort, constipation, or malabsorption.

Equally important is the vagus nerve's influence on sleep. Think of falling asleep as sinking gently into a quiet ocean, where waves of thought and tension gradually drift away. The vagus nerve plays a critical role in this transition by signaling the body to relax, helping regulate melatonin-the sleep hormone-and promoting deeper, more restorative rest. Quality sleep is not just about feeling refreshed; it supports memory, emotional regulation, and healing. When your vagus nerve is functioning optimally, it acts as a gatekeeper, gently guiding you into the deep, healing waters of sleep.

3.2 The Simple Science Behind the Vagus Nerve

Let's simplify how to tap into the power of the vagus nerve in your everyday life.

Imagine it's the end of a demanding day-you feel tense, fatigued, and mentally overloaded. Your nervous system is still in high alert. Now, with just a few intentional breaths, you can change that state. Deep, diaphragmatic breathing-inhaling slowly through your nose and exhaling gently through your mouth-activates the vagus nerve and shifts your body from fight-or-flight into rest-and-repair.

Other practices like gentle yoga, meditation, singing, humming, gargling, or even immersing your face in cold water can enhance vagal tone—the strength and responsiveness of the vagus nerve. These practices essentially tune your nervous system like a musical instrument, creating harmony in both body and mind.

Reflection Exercise: Finding Your Calm

Take a moment to reflect on a recent time when stress felt overwhelming. How did your body react? Were there physical sensations, like a racing heart or shallow breathing? Record these observations and consider incorporating practices that stimulate the vagus nerve into your daily routine. Which calming practices resonate with you? Can you commit to 5 minutes of deep breathing daily? A calming walk in nature? A quiet pause before bed? Whether it's a few minutes of deep breathing, a gentle yoga session, or a quiet moment of mindfulness, these practices can empower you to harness the vagus nerve's calming influence. Even small steps can build the foundation for nervous system resilience.

3.3 The Science Behind Vagus Nerve Function: A Simplified Overview

The vagus nerve has captivated scientists for its wide-ranging influence on health. As the longest cranial nerve, it connects the brain to major organs—including the heart, lungs, gut, and liver-playing acentral role in regulating involuntary bodily functions.

Recent neuroscience research has revealed that stimulating the vagus nerve not only affects physical functions like heart rate and digestion but also mental health. Clinical studies show that vagus nerve stimulation (VNS)-either invasive or non-invasive-can significantly reduce symptoms of treatment-resistant depression, anxiety, and epilepsy. This discovery has opened new therapeutic doors, especially for those who haven't responded to conventional medications.

Tools like heart rate variability (HRV) are now being used to measure vagal tone, offering a window into your nervous system's adaptability. Higher HRV indicates better vagal function and resilience to stress. With biofeedback and mindfulness-based techniques, individuals can learn to improve their HRV, thereby enhancing their ability to shift into calm states more efficiently.

However, mapping the vagus nerve's full complexity remains a scientific challenge. Imaging technologies like MRI and ultrasound can't yet fully capture its branching pathways and interactions with other nerves. Continued research into vagus nerve function, mapping, and stimulation is vital to unlocking its full healing potential.

3.4 The Vagus Nerve and Neuroplasticity

Your brain is not fixed-it's constantly rewiring and reshaping itself based on experiences. This ability, known as neuroplasticity, allows you to learn new things, recover from injury, and adapt emotionally. It's like a living map that redraws itself in response to life's journey.

The vagus nerve is a key player in this adaptive process. When stimulated, it can enhance the brain's ability to form new, healthier connections-especially in areas related to emotion, memory, and attention. That's why vagus nerve stimulation is being explored as a treatment for conditions like PTSD, stroke recovery, tinnitus, and chronic anxiety.

In individuals with depression or trauma, negative neural patterns can become "hardwired." VNS helps break those loops by encouraging flexibility and new circuits that support healing. It's as if the brain is being given a new route to travel-one paved with peace rather than fear.

Everyday practices like meditation, movement, breathwork, and even listening to calming music can gently stimulate the vagus nerve and promote neuroplasticity. Over time, these habits reshape your inner landscape, building emotional resilience and a more regulated nervous system.

3.5 What Is Polyvagal Theory?

Polyvagal Theory, developed by Dr. Stephen Porges, offers a groundbreaking framework to understand how the vagus nerve shapes your emotional and physiological states. Instead of viewing the autonomic nervous system with two opposite parts (fight-or-flight vs.rest-and-digest), this theory introduces a more nuanced, hierarchical model based on perceived safety.

The three primary states:

1. Ventral Vagal (Social Engagement State): When we feel safe, the ventral vagus is active. This supports calmness, facial expression, eye contact, and connection. It's the state where empathy, trust, and love flourish.
2. Sympathetic (Mobilization State): When we sense danger, the sympathetic nervous system takes over, preparing us to fight or flee. Our heart rate increases, muscles tense, and we become hyper-alert. This state is vital for survival, but chronic activation can lead to anxiety, panic, and burnout.
3. Dorsal Vagal (Shutdown State): When we experience extreme threat or trauma, the dorsal branch of the vagus nerve activates, causing collapse or freeze. We might feel numb, disconnected, dissociated, or hopeless. While

it's a protective mechanism, remaining stuck here can mimic depression and chronic fatigue.

Polyvagal Theory also introduces neuroception-the subconscious ability to detect cues of safety or threat in the environment. This internal surveillance system influences how we engage with others, regulate emotions, and respond to life's stressors. When neuroception misfires, it can lead to hypervigilance or withdrawal, even in safe environments.

In this chapter, we uncovered the vagus nerve's critical role in helping the body rest, digest, and sleep-core processes necessary for physical repair, emotional stability, and mental clarity. Acting as the body's internal conductor, the vagus nerve fine-tunes our physiological state, promoting calm, regulating digestion, improving sleep quality, and facilitating emotional resilience through neuroplasticity and the framework of Polyvagal Theory. Understanding how to activate and support this nerve can offer profound healing opportunities, especially in today's stress-laden world.

Now that we've explored the restorative potential of a well-functioning vagus nerve, it's important to recognize what happens when things go wrong. In the next chapter, we'll dive into the disruptions, dysfunctions, and imbalances that can affect the vagus nerve-and how these issues can manifest in chronic pain, inflammation, digestive disorders, mental health struggles, and more. By identifying the signs of vagal imbalance, we set the foundation for targeted healing strategies and natural interventions that bring the body back into balance.

Chapter 4: Disruptions, Dysfunction, & Imbalances of the Vagus Nerve

Picture yourself standing in the middle of a bustling city, the chaos of honking cars, blaring sirens, and hurried pedestrians surrounding you. This scene can resemble the internal storm our bodies endure when stress takes over, disrupting the delicate balance maintained by the vagus nerve. Our modern lives often resemble this city, with persistent demands pulling us in every direction, leaving little room for calm or rest. Amid this turmoil, the vagus nerve emerges as a beacon of hope, counterbalancing the relentless stress cycle. It is a vital component of the parasympathetic nervous system, offering a pathway back to tranquility and equilibrium.

4.1 The Vagus Nerve and the Stress Response

The vagus nerve is unique in its role in the body's stress response, acting as a moderator that helps the body navigate the complex stress landscape. When a stressful event occurs, the body's sympathetic nervous system is activated, triggering the fight-or-flight response. This reaction is essential for survival, preparing you to confront or escape danger. It floods your system with adrenaline, increasing heart rate and blood pressure, sharpening your senses, and redirecting blood flow to essential muscles. At this moment, the vagus nerve stands ready to restore balance, counteracting the effects of this heightened state. It signals the heart to slow down, encourages deep, steady breathing, and promotes relaxation, helping your body return to a state of calm.

Chronic stress, however, poses a significant threat to this balance, with lasting consequences for health and well-being. Persistent high levels of stress hormones can lead to issues such as chronic pain, anxiety, depression, difficulty concentrating, mood swings, and gut inflammation. Imagine stress as a constant barrage of traffic jams in the body, overwhelming the vagus nerve's ability to maintain order. Over time, this relentless pressure can lead to vagal dysfunction, diminishing the nerve's capacity to perform its crucial regulatory roles. The result can be a downward spiral of health issues, where stress begets more stress, creating a cycle that can be challenging to break.

Fortunately, specific techniques can activate the vagus nerve, helping mitigate stress's effects and restore balance. Simple practices such as deep, slow belly breathing can have a profound impact, encouraging the body to relax and recover. When you focus on taking slow, deliberate breaths, you engage the diaphragm, stimulating the vagus nerve and promoting a sense of calm and relaxation. Other methods include immersing your face in cold water, loudly gargling or singing, humming, and even laughing, all of which can activate the vagus nerve and support stress relief.

Case studies provide compelling evidence of the benefits of vagus nerve stimulation for stress management. For instance, people who have integrated these techniques into their daily routines often report significant improvements in mood, pain management, and overall well-being. One such case involved a patient of mine struggling with chronic anxiety who found relief through the regular practice of diaphragmatic breathing and cold exposure. Over time, these practices not only reduced anxiety levels but also enhanced resilience to stress, highlighting the transformative potential of vagus nerve modulation.

<u>*Reflection: Identifying Stress Triggers*</u>

Take a moment to reflect on the stressors in your life. What situations or events trigger your stress response? Are there patterns or common themes? Consider keeping a journal to track these triggers and your body's reactions. By identifying these patterns, you can become more aware of how stress affects your vagus nerve and explore techniques to maintain calmness and balance in challenging situations. This awareness is the first step toward harnessing the power of the vagus nerve to enhance your well-being.

4.2 What Common Factors Lead to Vagal Imbalance

Navigating the complexities of life, it's not uncommon to encounter overwhelming stress. This stress, when prolonged, can strain the vagus nerve, causing it to become imbalanced. Imagine carrying a heavy backpack every day; eventually, the weight wears you down. Similarly, stress overload taxes your nervous system, hampering its ability to regulate bodily functions effectively. The trauma experienced by a person compounds this effect, whether from a sudden event or sustained hardship. It leaves a mark, disrupting the nerve's ability to communicate smoothly across the body's systems. Physical trauma might seem obvious, like a car accident leaving a lingering physical impact. Yet, emotional trauma can be just as profound, often more challenging to pinpoint, but equally disruptive. The scars of past experiences can obstruct the vagus nerve's pathways, creating roadblocks to overall healing and well-being.

A sedentary lifestyle adds another layer of complexity. In today's digital age, it's easy to fall into patterns of inactivity. Hours spent sitting at a desk or lounging on the couch contribute to decreased vagal tone. Movement is a natural stimulant for the vagus nerve; it's like oil for an engine, keeping everything running smoothly. Without it, the body becomes sluggish, and the nerve loses vitality. Coupled with poor sleep, which deprives the body of essential repair time, the cumulative effects can be profound. Sleep is when the nervous system resets, processing the day's events and restoring balance. Inadequate rest, characterized by restless nights or insufficient sleep, leaves the body in a constant state of catch-up, stressing the vagus nerve.

The diet also plays a pivotal role. Unhealthy eating habits, rich in processed foods and low in essential nutrients, deprive the body of what it needs to support nerve health. Imagine fueling a car with low-grade gasoline; eventually, the engine suffers. Chronic inflammation, often associated with diet, can lead to further deterioration. It's the body's way of signaling distress, a fire that, if left unchecked, can cause lasting damage. Infections fuel this fire, taxing the immune system and, by extension, the vagus nerve, which is integrally connected to the immune response.

Anxiety and depression are both causes and effects of vagal imbalance. They create a feedback loop where the nerve's compromised state exacerbates these conditions and vice versa. Social isolation compounds these feelings, depriving the body of the regulating effects of social interaction. Human connection stimulates the vagus nerve, promoting a sense of safety and well-being. Without it, the nerve's tone weakens, furthering the cycle of imbalance. Surgeries, while often necessary, pose risks to nerve function. The body interprets surgery as trauma, responding with inflammation and stress, both of which strain the vagus nerve.

The aging process naturally affects the nervous system, including the vagus nerve. Like any part of the body, it can lose efficiency over time. Environmental toxins, from pollutants to chemicals in everyday products, introduce additional stressors. They infiltrate the body, creating a toxic load that the nervous system must work overtime to manage. Though beneficial in many ways, medications can have side effects that alter nerve function. Lastly, unresolved grief or emotional suppression acts like an invisible weight, burdening the nerve and preventing it from functioning optimally. Each factor, on its own, may seem manageable, but together, they create a tapestry of challenges that can lead to significant vagal imbalance.

4.3 Symptoms and Conditions You Could Experience with Vagus Nerve Dysfunction

Imagine waking up one morning feeling overwhelmed by anxiety, your mind racing, and your heart pounding before you've even begun the day. Although distressing, this sensation is a common experience for individuals with vagus nerve dysfunction. The vagus nerve, a key player in regulating mood, can significantly influence your emotional state. When its function is compromised, you might find yourself more susceptible to heightened anxiety, frequent mood swings, or even depression. These mood disorders can feel like a rollercoaster of emotions, where the highs and lows disrupt your daily life and relationships. It's as if the very foundation of your emotional stability is shaken, leaving you searching for calm amidst the chaos.

The digestive system, often called the body's "second brain," is another area profoundly affected by vagus nerve dysfunction. As we discussed earlier, you might experience persistent digestive issues, such as bloating, gas, or discomfort, which can interfere with your ability to enjoy meals or feel nourished. For example, this dysfunction can lead to conditions like Irritable Bowel Syndrome (IBS), where the gut's communication with the brain becomes erratic, causing symptoms like abdominal pain or irregular bowel habits. Imagine feeling constantly on edge, anticipating when the next wave of discomfort will hit, disrupting your daily routine and diminishing your quality of life. These digestive challenges can become persistent, affecting your physical and emotional well-being.

Chronic pain is another symptom that can arise from vagus nerve dysfunction, manifesting as persistent aches or discomfort in various parts of the body. This pain can be both physically and mentally exhausting, coloring your days with a backdrop of unease. It can be challenging to pinpoint the exact cause of this pain, as it often results from the nerve's impaired ability to regulate inflammation and pain perception. Living with chronic pain can feel like an uphill battle, where each day requires more effort and resilience to push through the discomfort and maintain a semblance of normalcy.

Heart irregularities can also occur when the vagus nerve's function is compromised, leading to episodes of palpitations or an irregular heartbeat. These symptoms can be unsettling, causing you to worry about your heart's health and overall well-being. The vagus nerve plays a crucial role in moderating heart rate. When its signals are disrupted, you may feel anxious and uncertain about the stability of your cardiovascular system. This irregularity can create a lingering sense of unease, as if your body's rhythm is out of sync with the world around you.

Breathing is another vital function regulated by the vagus nerve, and dysfunction can lead to lung-related symptoms, such as shortness of breath or difficulty breathing deeply. These symptoms can feel like a weight on your chest, making it challenging to find the breath you need to feel calm and centered. Sleep, essential for restoration and rejuvenation, can also be disrupted by vagus nerve dysfunction, leading to sleep disorders such as insomnia or restless sleep. Without restorative rest, you may be caught in a cycle of fatigue and irritability, where the day's demands feel insurmountable.

Finally, Postural Orthostatic Tachycardia Syndrome (POTS) is associated with vagus nerve dysfunction, characterized by an abnormal increase in heart rate and a decrease in blood pressure when transitioning from lying to standing. This dysfunction can cause dizziness, lightheadedness, and even fainting, making daily activities a daunting challenge. POTS can feel like your body is betraying you, leaving you struggling to maintain balance and confidence in your movements. These symptoms underscore the critical role of the vagus nerve in maintaining balance and well-being, highlighting the complex interplay between physiological and emotional health.

4.4 How the Feedback Loop of the Vagus Nerve Malfunctions and Dysregulation Spirals

Picture the vagus nerve as the body's internal communication highway, tasked with maintaining equilibrium by relaying vital information between the brain and body. It's like a finely tuned orchestra, where each section must play harmoniously to keep the music flowing. When the vagus nerve functions well, it helps regulate stress responses, digestion, immune function, and emotional health. However, stress and illness can throw this system off balance, depleting the nerve's ability to perform its duties. Imagine a conductor who struggles to guide the orchestra, overwhelmed by external noise. The result is a cacophony, where the instruments no longer play in sync, and the melody is lost. This loss of harmony in the body manifests as a malfunctioning feedback loop, where signals that should bring calm and balance become distorted or drowned out by chaos.

As stress or illness persists, the impaired feedback loop exacerbates the issue, compounding the stress and leading to further depletion of the vagus nerve function. It's a vicious cycle, like a snowball gathering momentum downhill, growing more significant and unmanageable with each turn. The nerve, overwhelmed by constant demands, struggles to send clear signals, causing a cascade of effects throughout the body. The immune system, intricately linked to the vagus nerve, becomes less responsive, leaving the body vulnerable to infections and chronic inflammation. This ongoing inflammation acts like a persistent fire, damaging tissues and organs and further straining the body's resources. As the body's defenses falter, the mind and emotions also suffer, leading to increased anxiety, mood swings, and even depression.

This spiral of dysregulation impacts mental and emotional health profoundly. Imagine navigating a rural mountain road in the dark without headlights; without light and clear guidance, the road becomes fraught with obstacles and uncertainty. The vagus nerve acts as a beacon, guiding the body through stress and restoring balance when functioning optimally.

But when it's compromised, that guidance fades, leaving the nervous system reactive and oversensitive. Emotional resilience decreases, and minor stressors become overwhelming challenges. The body's ability to cope with life's ups and downs diminishes, leaving you feeling exhausted and on edge. It's as if the body's internal compass is misaligned, unable to point you toward calm and well-being.

The interplay between stress, inflammation, and vagal dysfunction creates a complex web that can be difficult to untangle. Yet, understanding this connection empowers you to recognize the signs of imbalance and take steps to restore harmony. You can repair this feedback loop by nurturing the vagus nerve, promoting resilience and healing. Simple practices, like mindful breathing, gentle movement, and fostering connections, can help reignite the vagus nerve's ability to guide the body toward balance. As the feedback loop strengthens, the body's systems can return to a state of coherence, where stress is managed effectively, inflammation is kept in check, and emotional health is restored. It's a gradual process, like the slow return of spring after a long, frigid winter; restoring this feedback loop takes time—but the light of well-being will shine again.

4.5 The Ripple Effect

Imagine your body as a finely tuned orchestra, each system playing its part in creating a symphony of health. The vagus nerve is the conductor, ensuring harmony among the cardiovascular, digestive, immune, and endocrine systems. When the vagus nerve functions optimally, it helps maintain balance, allowing each system to perform its role seamlessly. However, this balance is disrupted when dysfunction occurs, creating a ripple effect that resonates throughout the body.

Remember that the vagus nerve plays a crucial role in cardiovascular health, regulating heart rate and blood pressure. It acts like a brake, slowing down the heart rate when necessary and helping to maintain a steady rhythm. When the vagus nerve is compromised, its ability to regulate these functions diminishes, leading to irregular heartbeats or elevated blood pressure. This disruption can increase the risk of cardiovascular issues, such as heart disease or hypertension. The heart, no longer receiving the calming signals it needs, may work harder than it should, creating strain on the cardiovascular system over time.

The ripple effect extends to the digestive system, where the vagus nerve is vital in regulating digestion and nutrient absorption. It stimulates the production of digestive enzymes and controls muscle contractions that move food through the gastrointestinal tract. Digestion proceeds smoothly when the vagus nerve functions well, ensuring nutrients are absorbed efficiently. However, when its function is impaired, digestive processes can become erratic, leading to symptoms like bloating, discomfort, or irregular bowel movements. The body's ability to extract nutrients from food diminishes, affecting overall health and vitality.

In the realm of the immune system, the vagus nerve influences the body's inflammatory response. It helps modulate the production of cytokines, proteins that signal immune cells to act. When the vagus nerve is balanced, it prevents excessive inflammation, protecting tissues from damage. However, this regulatory function falters when it becomes dysfunctional, leading to chronic inflammation. This ongoing inflammation acts like an out-of-tune instrument, contributing to the development of autoimmune conditions and other inflammatory disorders. Instead of protecting the body, the defense mechanisms may inadvertently cause harm, further straining the immune system.

The endocrine system, responsible for hormone production and regulation, is also affected by vagus nerve dysfunction. This nerve helps coordinate the release of hormones that regulate stress, metabolism, and mood. When the vagus nerve is functioning well, it ensures that hormones are released in appropriate amounts, maintaining balance and stability. However, hormone levels may fluctuate when its function is impaired, leading to imbalances that affect mood, energy levels, and metabolic processes. This disruption can manifest as fatigue, mood swings, or weight changes, impacting overall well-being.

The ripple effect of vagus nerve dysfunction underscores the interconnectedness of the body's systems and its impact on overall health. Each system relies on the vagus nerve for regulation and balance, and the consequences of dysfunction are far-reaching. By understanding how imbalances manifest, we can better appreciate the importance of maintaining vagal health, as it holds the key to preserving the harmony and balance that underpins overall well-being. By nurturing the vagus nerve, we can support the body's ability to adapt, heal, and thrive, fostering a resilient foundation for health. This understanding sets the stage for the next chapter, which explores and addresses your vagal imbalances and provides strategies to address them, empowering you to reclaim your vitality and well-being.

Conclusion

Understanding the critical role of the vagus nerve in our body's ability to rest, digest, and sleep provides a powerful foundation for holistic healing. From regulating heart rate and digestion to calming the mind and supporting restorative sleep, the vagus nerve is intricately tied to our physical, emotional, and mental well-being. When we learn to stimulate and support this vital nerve pathway, we open the door to improved resilience, reduced stress, and a greater sense of balance in our daily lives.

But what happens when this nerve is not functioning optimally? In the next chapter, we'll explore how to recognize the signs and symptoms of vagus nerve imbalance, how it can manifest in various health conditions, and why understanding your personal vagus nerve function is key to restoring full-body harmony.

STEP TWO

ASSESS YOUR VAGUS POWER

Chapter 5: Is Your Vagus Nerve Imbalanced?

Imagine waking up each morning feeling like you're carrying an invisible 50-pound weight. Your body feels sluggish, your mind is foggy, and you're navigating through the day with an inexplicable sense of unease. These feelings might seem like a typical scenario of stress or fatigue, but it could be your body's way of signaling an imbalance in your vagus nerve. Just as a car needs regular maintenance to run smoothly, your vagus nerve requires attention to ensure it functions optimally. This chapter introduces the concept of self-assessment for vagus nerve health, a crucial step toward understanding and addressing any imbalances you may be experiencing.

5.1 Self-Assessment

Self-assessment can be daunting, especially involving something as intricate as the vagus nerve. However, taking a closer look at your health is empowering. It enables you to gain insights into how your body functions and identify areas that need attention. A self-assessment is a diagnostic tool that offers a snapshot of your vagal health. It guides you in recognizing patterns and understanding how factors-such as stress, diet, and lifestyle-impact your overall well-being. Regularly evaluating your health makes you more attuned to your body's signals, enabling you to make informed decisions about your care.

One of the most effective ways to engage in self-assessment is through journaling. Daily tracking of your health metrics can provide valuable insights into your vagal health over time. Consider tracking your mood, energy levels, sleep quality, and digestion. Not only does this practice help you identify patterns and triggers, but it also allows you to measure improvements as you implement changes. Journaling encourages mindfulness, fostering a deeper connection with your body and helping you recognize subtle shifts in your health. Over time, these observations can guide you in fine-tuning your lifestyle and interventions to support vagus nerve balance.

Interactive Element: Journaling Prompts for Vagal Health

Begin by setting aside a few minutes daily to journal about your health and well-being. Use the following prompts to guide your reflections:

1. *How did you sleep last night? Did you wake up feeling refreshed or fatigued?*

2. *What was your mood like today? Did you feel calm, anxious, or somewhere in between?*

3. *How were your energy levels throughout the day? Did you experience any highs or lows?*

4. *How was your digestion today? Did you experience any discomfort or irregularity?*

5. *What activities or events seemed to impact your mood or energy today?*

Regularly engaging with these prompts creates a personal log that reveals trends and insights into your vagal health. This practice helps you monitor your progress and empowers you to take proactive steps toward enhancing your well-being. Recognizing and addressing imbalances in your vagus nerve is a journey of self-discovery and empowerment, offering profound transformation and healing potential.

5.2 The Vagus Nerve Depletion Quiz

When understanding your health, having a clear picture of your vagus nerve function can be invaluable. The Vagus Nerve Depletion Quiz is a straightforward yet insightful tool designed to help you assess the current state of your vagal health. It is a check-in to gauge how well your vagus nerve supports your overall well-being. This quiz covers various aspects of your health, from physical symptoms to emotional well-being, providing a comprehensive overview of potential imbalances. By answering a series of questions, you can better understand how your lifestyle and experiences may impact this vital nerve. The quiz is structured to be user-friendly, utilizing a simple scoring system that makes interpretation easy, empowering you to take proactive steps toward balance.

The quiz consists of 20 questions, each focusing on a different aspect of your health. For each question, rate your experience on a scale from 0 to 4, where 0= "Never," 1= "Rarely," 2= "Sometimes," 3= "Often," and 4= "Always." These questions are designed to cover a range of symptoms and feelings, offering a holistic view of your vagal health. So, get something to record your answers with.

VAGUS NERVE DEPLETION QUIZ

Section 1: Physical Symptoms

1. I frequently feel bloated, constipated, or experience digestive issues like IBS.

2. My heart feels irregular, or I often feel my heartbeat racing without exerting myself.

3. I get dizzy or lightheaded when standing up too quickly.

4. I experience frequent headaches or migraines.

5. My throat often feels tight, or I have difficulty swallowing without a physical cause.

Section 2: Emotional Well-being

1. I often feel stressed, worried, or overwhelmed.
2. I have difficulty calming down after feeling upset or agitated.
3. I experience frequent feelings of low mood or depression.
4. I feel socially withdrawn or struggle to connect with others emotionally.
5. I have a poor ability to cope with minor inconveniences or challenges.

Section 3: Sleep and Fatigue

1. I often feel tired or fatigued, even after a whole night's sleep.
2. I have trouble falling or staying asleep.
3. I wake up feeling groggy or unrefreshed most mornings
4. My body often feels tense or restless at night
5. I clench my jaw, grind my teeth, or feel tense while sleeping.

Section 4: Immune and Inflammation Symptoms

1. I frequently get sick or take longer than usual to recover from illness.

2. I often experience inflammation, such as joint pain, swelling, or puffiness.

3. I notice increased allergies or sensitivities to environmental, animal, or food triggers.

4. I experience chronic pain or discomfort in my body.

5. I have a history of inflammatory or autoimmune conditions.

Scoring And Interpretation

You've taken a big step in taking this quiz, and because you answered these questions honestly, you can identify patterns that may be impacting your vagus nerve. After completing the quiz, tally your scores to understand where you stand. A higher score suggests a greater likelihood of vagus nerve depletion, while a lower score indicates a healthier vagal tone.

Your Score: __________

0-20: Strong Vagal tone; you're likely managing your stress and have strong resilience.

21-40: Mild vagus nerve depletion; consider incorporating vagus nerve stimulation techniques.

41-60: Moderate depletion; prioritize your daily activities and habits that strengthen your vagal tone. You should seek help from a healthcare professional to get support.

61-80: Severe depletion; you must consult a healthcare professional for personalized treatment strategies.

Regular assessment is crucial for tracking changes in your vagal health over time. Just as you wouldn't expect to plant a garden and never tend to it, your health requires ongoing attention and care. Consider retaking the quiz every few weeks or months, depending on the severity of your depletion. You can also re-test whenever you notice significant changes in your symptoms or lifestyle. This periodic evaluation allows you to monitor progress, noting improvements and areas requiring extra attention. By maintaining this awareness, you can make informed adjustments to your habits and routines, fostering a supportive environment for your vagus nerve.

As you reflect on your quiz results, take a moment to consider the factors contributing to your scores. Look at your lifestyle, stress levels, diet, and sleep patterns. Are there areas where you could introduce positive changes? Incorporating more relaxation techniques or improving sleep hygiene could be beneficial. Use your reflections to guide and help you prioritize areas of your life that may need extra care. Remember, your goal is not perfection but progress. By understanding the needs of your vagus nerve, you empower yourself to make choices that support your health and well-being. This powerful self-awareness tool enables you to take control of your health with confidence and compassion.

5.3 How to Rebalance Your Vagus Nerve

Rebalancing your vagus nerve begins with nurturing your body through lifestyle changes. The type and quality of foods you eat are pivotal in this. Think of nutrition as fuel, not just for your muscles but also for your nervous system. A diet rich in whole foods, like leafy greens, lean proteins, and healthy fats, supports your body's needs and reduces inflammation. Cutting down on processed foods and sugars can help alleviate stress on your body, promoting a more balanced nerve function.

Exercise is another cornerstone of vagal health. It doesn't have to be intense; consistency is key. Daily walks, gentle yoga, or swimming can boost your mood and enhance your vagal tone. Exercise stimulates the release of endorphins, which naturally elevates your sense of well-being and, over time, improves your body's resilience to stress. Sleep hygiene, often overlooked, is equally vital. Establish a routine prioritizing rest, aiming for seven to nine hours of quality sleep. A regular sleep schedule supports the circadian (24-hour) rhythm, which helps regulate the vagus nerve. Reducing exposure to toxins is also crucial. These toxins include not only environmental toxins but also limiting alcohol and caffeine, which can stress the nervous system.

Incorporating mind-body practices can dramatically enhance vagal tone. Yoga and Tai Chi are excellent for promoting relaxation and flexibility, both physically and mentally. These disciplines encourage slow, mindful movements and deep breathing, which engage the vagus nerve. Meditation and mindfulness practices help anchor you in the present, reducing stress and anxiety. Simple breathing exercises, for example, inhaling deeply through the nose and exhaling slowly through the mouth, can be practiced anywhere and effectively calm the nervous system. Hydrotherapy (using water as a treatment therapy) benefits the vagus nerve. Try alternating hot and cold water for your body. Research has shown that cold exposure activates the vagus nerve, enhancing its function and boosting overall resilience. So, dipping your face in cool water, taking or ending your shower with cool water, or taking a cool plunge can invigorate and activate the vagus nerve.

Therapeutic approaches offer additional support for vagus nerve health, especially if you're dealing with trauma or chronic stress. Counseling provides a safe space for exploring emotional challenges and developing effective coping strategies. Trauma therapy, including Eye Movement Desensitization and Reprocessing (EMDR) and Somatic Experiencing, focuses on releasing trapped energy in the body, helping to restore balance. These therapies work by gently guiding you through traumatic memories, allowing the nervous system to process and integrate these experiences.

Vagus nerve stimulation (VNS) is a new area of research. VNS can complement these therapies through devices that send impulses directly to the vagus nerve from a device implanted under your skin. You can also use external devices, many of which are now on the market, but beware that many have not been tested for safety and effectiveness. Finally, you can use the previously discussed techniques to relieve your symptoms and promote healing. We will discuss more about VNS in the next chapter.

Social engagement is a powerful yet often underestimated component of vagus nerve health. Building and maintaining positive relationships provides emotional support and fosters a sense of belonging. Engage in activities that bring you joy and connect you with others, whether volunteering, joining groups or clubs, or simply spending time with loved ones. Meaningful social interactions stimulate the vagus nerve, enhancing its ability to regulate emotions and stress responses. This aspect of vagal health underscores the interconnection between our emotional and physical well-being. A warm hug, a shared laugh, or a heartfelt conversation can nourish your nervous system like a balanced diet or regular exercise.

5.4 Activating Parasympathetic Response: Techniques for Daily Calm

Imagine your life as a series of balancing acts, constantly shifting between moments of stress and calm. In this dynamic dance, activating the parasympathetic response is like finding your center, a space where you can breathe deeply and feel grounded. The vagus nerve plays a crucial role here, as it's the key player in the parasympathetic nervous system, promoting relaxation and recovery. Regularly engaging in this response allows your body to rest, digest, and heal, counterbalancing the hectic pace of modern life. It's like pressing a reset button, allowing you to approach challenges with renewed clarity and resilience.

One effective technique to stimulate the vagus nerve is progressive muscle relaxation. This process involves systematically tensing and releasing different muscle groups, starting from your toes and working your way up to your head. As you do this, focus on the sensation of relaxation spreading through your body, like a wave of calm washing over you. This practice activates the vagus nerve, helping to release physical tension and fostering a sense of peace. Another method is mindful meditation, where you focus on your breath, observing each inhalation and exhalation without judgment or attachment. By centering your attention on the present moment, you engage the vagus nerve, encouraging a state of tranquility and balance. Many free and inexpensive apps are available to learn how to meditate. Meditation may seem strange, but the research shows its effectiveness.

I cannot overstate the benefits of consistency in these practices. Just as a musician improves with daily practice, your body becomes more adept at accessing the parasympathetic response with regular engagement. Over time, these exercises can profoundly change your stress levels and overall well-being. By incorporating them into your daily routine, you cultivate a habit of calmness, enabling you to navigate life's ups and downs with greater ease. This commitment to regular practice is an investment in your health, offering far-reaching, long-term benefits beyond immediate stress relief.

Consider the story of Jessica, a busy professional who felt perpetually overwhelmed by her demanding job. She began incorporating deep breathing exercises and progressive muscle relaxation into her daily routine. Initially skeptical, she soon noticed a shift in her stress levels. Taking a few moments each day to focus on her breath and release tension transformed her outlook. Jessica was more present and less reactive, with a clearer mind and a lighter mood. Her experience serves as a testament to the power of these techniques, demonstrating how engaging the parasympathetic response can foster resilience and overall well-being.

For easy-to-implement strategies, start with something as simple as diaphragmatic breathing. Sit comfortably, placing one hand on your chest and the other on your abdomen. Slowly breathe through your nose, allowing your stomach to expand. Exhale through your mouth, feeling the gentle contraction of your abdominal muscles. When practiced for a few minutes daily, this exercise can significantly enhance vagal tone, reduce stress, and promote relaxation. These small steps, integrated into daily life, can lead to meaningful change, helping you cultivate a sense of calm and balance amidst the chaos.

5.5 Heart Rate Variability Unpacked

Heart Rate Variability (HRV) may sound technical, but it's essentially a measure of the variation in time between each heartbeat. This variability reflects the autonomic nervous system's balance, particularly the vagus nerve's influence. A healthy heart doesn't beat like a metronome but adjusts its rhythm in response to your body's needs. This adaptability, or variability, is a sign of resilience. When your vagal tone is strong, your HRV is higher, indicating that your body can efficiently switch between states of rest and activity. This flexibility is closely tied to how well you handle stress and is a powerful predictor of overall health. A robust HRV suggests that your heart can quickly adapt to stressors, promoting long-term cardiovascular health and reducing the risk of chronic diseases.

Measuring HRV is surprisingly accessible with today's technology. Many wearable devices, like smartwatches and fitness trackers, offer HRV monitoring as a feature. These devices often sync with smartphone apps, providing a detailed analysis of your heart's variability at your fingertips. Measuring your HRV is simple. Wear the device as instructed, typically on your wrist, and allow it to collect data over a specified period. Apps like Elite HRV, Wellatory, or HRV4Training are popular for tracking and interpreting your HRV data if you don't have a smartwatch or fitness tracker. These apps use the camera on your phone. They can provide daily readings and trends, helping you understand how stress, sleep, and lifestyle choices impact your vagal health. Regularly monitoring your HRV offers valuable insights into your body's response to various stimuli and can help you make informed decisions to enhance your overall well-being.

At first, understanding HRV results can be overwhelming, but it's pretty straightforward. Generally, a higher HRV is associated with a healthier autonomic nervous system and better vagal tone. It reflects your body's ability to adapt to stress and recover efficiently. Conversely, a lower HRV may indicate stress, fatigue, or potential health issues. Tracking your HRV over time enables you to identify patterns and trends correlating with lifestyle events or changes. For example, you may notice a dip in HRV after a stressful week, indicating how stress affects your health. This awareness allows you to connect the dots between your lifestyle and your body's responses, empowering you to make targeted adjustments.

Improving your HRV is about nurturing your vagus nerve through intentional practices. Again, regular meditation sessions focusing on deep, rhythmic breathing can enhance vagal activity and HRV. Engaging in activities like Tai Chi or Qigong, which combine movement with mindfulness, can also bolster your heart's variability. These practices promote relaxation and balance, allowing your autonomic nervous system to function optimally. Additionally, incorporating physical exercise, maintaining good sleep hygiene, and fostering positive social connections can all contribute to a healthier HRV.

To illustrate the impact of HRV monitoring, consider the story of Jacob, an amateur athlete who wanted to improve his performance. By tracking his HRV, he discovered that his variability was lower than expected, often correlating with periods of intense training and inadequate rest. Recognizing this, Jacob adjusted his routine to include more recovery days and focused on stress-reduction techniques. Over time, his HRV improved, and he noticed increased stamina and reduced anxiety during competitions. Jacob's experience highlights the potential of HRV monitoring as a tool for personal growth and health optimization. By understanding and acting on these insights, you can also enhance your physical and emotional resilience.

As you've discovered in this chapter, understanding the state of your vagus nerve through self-assessment and practical tools like journaling and heart rate variability monitoring empowers you to take control of your well-being. But awareness is just the beginning. Now that you've gained insight into how an imbalanced vagus nerve can affect your body, it's time to turn inward and explore its profound influence on your mental and emotional landscape. The next chapter builds on this foundation, guiding you through the intricate connection between the vagus nerve and your emotional health. From stress and anxiety to trauma and depression, we'll dive into how your vagus nerve shapes your inner world—and how to nurture it to cultivate calm, clarity, and emotional resilience.

I'd Love Your Honest Feedback So Far!

Hi there,

Thank you for reading the first part of ***Rebalance Your Vagus Nerve Superhighway: The Ultimate 3-Step Strategic Roadmap to Relieve Pain, Calm your Mind, Improve Sleep, and Restore Gut Health*** by **Dr. Kerri L. Jones, N.M.D.**

I know it might seem a little unusual to ask for a review before you've finished the entire book—but I'd truly love to hear your honest thoughts while everything is still fresh in your mind. Sometimes, we get to the end of a book and forget to share how it impacted us along the way.

Even if you're only halfway through, your perspective matters.

Whether you've already learned something new, started making small changes, or simply feel more hopeful and empowered, your voice can help others who are looking for support with stress, pain, digestion, trauma, or emotional health.

Why Your Review Matters:

• It helps others discover this book when they need it most

• It tells bookstores and platforms that this book is worth sharing

• It encourages Dr. Kerri to keep writing more helpful books

How to Leave a Review:

Scan the QR code or click the link below to go directly to the review page:

https://www.amazon.com/review/review-your-purchases/?asin=1968147012

Then, just write a few simple thoughts, such as:

- What you've learned or liked so far
- How it's already helping you
- Who you recommend it to

Feel free to add a picture with your review too!
You could snap a photo of the book cover, your favorite page, or where you're reading—it really helps others connect with the book in a personal way.

Your review doesn't have to be long or detailed—just honest and from the heart.

You Matter—Your Healing Matters.

Thank you again for being part of this healing journey. Just like your vagus nerve carries signals between your body and brain, **your feedback helps guide us—and others—toward hope and healing.**

With gratitude and care,

Dr. Kerri L. Jones, N.M.D.
DrKerriPublishing@gmail.com
HypermobileDr.com

P.S. If you have enjoyed this book so far, get my next book in this series, "***Unleash Your Vagus Nerve Superhighway Potential: Explore Holistic Therapies for Nervous System Repair and Balance, Emotional Resilience, Immune Support, and Vital Energy Restoration***". This book discusses my specific recommendations and prescriptions to help you formulate your own plan for life-long healing.

STEP THREE

REBALANCE & OPTIMIZE YOUR BODY & LIFE

Chapter 6: Enhance Your Mental-Emotional Health through the Vagus Nerve

Imagine a serene lake, its surface undisturbed by wind or ripples. This image represents emotional regulation at its finest-a state where you feel balanced and calm, capable of gracefully weathering life's storms. Emotional regulation is the ability to maintain inner peace and tranquility by constructively managing and responding to emotions. The vagus nerve is crucial in this process and helps modulate your body's stress responses, ensuring that feelings don't overwhelm you. The vagus nerve supports emotional resilience and stability by balancing the autonomic nervous system, particularly enhancing parasympathetic activity.

6.1 Physiological and Emotional Regulation and Health

Let's review what we have learned so far. The physiological and emotional regulation process involves complex interactions within your body, with the vagus nerve as the conductor. When you encounter stress, your body releases a surge of stress hormones, preparing you for action. Next, the vagus nerve steps in, encouraging your heart rate to slow down and your breathing to deepen, returning you to a state of equilibrium. Vagal tone, the measure of vagus nerve activity, plays a pivotal role here. A high vagal tone is associated with greater emotional stability, enhancing your ability to recover from stress and regulate emotions. Additionally, the vagus nerve influences neurotransmitter levels, such as serotonin and dopamine, which affect mood and emotional well-being.

Recognizing key emotional health indicators can provide insight into the condition of your vagus nerve. For instance, persistent anxiety and stress may indicate a vagal imbalance as your body struggles to regulate its responses. Emotional numbness or detachment, where you feel disconnected from your feelings, also suggests vagal dysfunction.

Research shows that individuals with mood disorders like Attention Deficit Hyperactive Disorder (ADHD), Post-traumatic Stress Disorder (PTSD), Autism Spectrum Disorder (ASD), Borderline Personality Disorder (BPD), Obsessive Compulsive Disorder (OCD), and schizophrenia often exhibit lower heart rate variability (HRV) and vagal tone. Improving these imbalances through vagal stimulation can offer relief and support emotional health.

Recent research highlights the connection between emotional regulation and vagal function. Studies indicate that vagus nerve stimulation (VNS) can alleviate mood disorders by enhancing vagal tone. VNS promotes neuroplasticity, allowing your brain to form new connections that improve emotional responses. For instance, individuals with depression who receive VNS experience better mood regulation because the vagus nerve helps balance neurotransmitter levels. This evidence underscores the vagus nerve's potential to transform emotional health, offering a pathway to resilience.

Consider incorporating specific practices into your routine to enhance emotional regulation through vagus nerve stimulation. Mindful body scanning, a technique that focuses attention on different body parts, can help you become more aware of physical sensations and emotional states. This practice encourages relaxation and strengthens the vagal tone. Visualization techniques, where you imagine calming scenes or experiences, can also engage the vagus nerve, promoting emotional balance. Visualizing serene landscapes or envisioning positive outcomes activates your parasympathetic nervous system, fostering a sense of calm and well-being.

Visual Element: Emotional Regulation Checklist

Create a checklist to track your progress in emotional regulation. Include practices like mindful body scanning and visualization, noting when and how often you engage in them. Assess key emotional health indicators like stress levels and mood stability to gauge improvements. This checklist can guide your journey toward optimal emotional health, helping you identify effective strategies and celebrate progress.

6.2 Overcoming Anxiety: Vagus Nerve Techniques for Mental Clarity

Anxiety, a shared experience, is often rooted in physiological processes that can be traced back to vagus nerve functioning. The vagus nerve significantly influences the body's response to stress, and when it doesn't function properly, it can exacerbate anxiety symptoms. When the vagus nerve is dysregulated, it can lead to an increased heart rate, shallow breathing, and a heightened state of alertness. This alert state is the body's fight-or-flight mechanism kicking in, even when no immediate danger exists. It's as if your body is on high alert, ready to react to threats that might not even exist. This state can leave you feeling tense and on edge, with your nervous system struggling to find a sense of calm.

To alleviate anxiety, engaging the vagus nerve through specific exercises can be incredibly effective. Gentle neck stretches can release tension accumulated in the muscles, promoting relaxation. Imagine standing or sitting comfortably, gently tilting your head from side to side, and feeling the stretch along your neck. This simple movement encourages blood flow and can help activate the vagus nerve, calming your mind. Tapping techniques, where you gently tap areas like your cheeks or collarbone, can stimulate the vagus nerve. These tapping techniques are rooted in acupressure and encourage the body's natural relaxation response. Physical exercise, such as walking or cycling, is another powerful method. These activities stimulate the vagus nerve and enhance its tone, helping you achieve mental clarity and reduce anxiety.

Lifestyle changes play a crucial role in managing anxiety through the vagus nerve. A balanced diet rich in omega-3 fatty acids in foods like salmon and walnuts supports brain health and vagal function. Ensuring adequate sleep is equally essential, as rest allows the body to repair and reset, fostering a more resilient nervous system. Regular exercise not only improves cardiovascular health but also boosts endorphin levels, promoting a sense of well-being and reducing anxiety.

Real-life stories highlight the transformative power of these practices. Meet Emily, who struggled with overwhelming anxiety that affected her daily life. By integrating gentle neck stretches and a consistent walking routine, she noticed a significant reduction in her anxiety levels. Expert insights also support these techniques. Dr. John Smith, a neurologist, notes that engaging the vagus nerve can enhance parasympathetic activity, promoting a sense of calm and reducing anxiety. Through these approaches, individuals like Emily have found relief, achieved mental clarity, and reclaimed their lives from the grip of anxiety.

6.3 Chronic Stress and Fatigue

Chronic stress is like living in a constant state of emergency, where the body is perpetually prepared for either fight or flight. This relentless tension profoundly impacts the vagus nerve, diminishing its ability to engage the parasympathetic system—the branch responsible for rest and recovery. As stress persists, cortisol, the stress hormone, floods the body, creating a ripple effect that disrupts the delicate balance of your autonomic nervous system. Heart rate variability (HRV), remember that this is a measure of the variation in time between each heartbeat, becomes erratic, reflecting the underlying turmoil. This disruption leaves the vagus nerve struggling to maintain its vital role as the mediator of calm and balance, like a conductor unable to bring harmony to an orchestra's off-tune, chaotic performance.

The consequences of this imbalance manifest in various ways. You might find yourself enduring unexplained heart palpitations, where it feels like your heart is skipping a beat or racing without reason. Breathlessness, often mistaken for a physical ailment, can arise as your body struggles to regulate its breath under stress. Hyperventilation, where rapid, shallow breathing takes over, further exacerbates feelings of anxiety and panic. This cycle of stress and fatigue feeds into itself, creating a looping feedback of physical symptoms that can leave you feeling trapped and overwhelmed. It's a state of being on edge, where your body seems to operate on high alert, even in the absence of immediate danger, leading to exhaustion that seeps into both body and mind.

Breaking free from this cycle requires intentional strategies to restore balance and calm. Utilize any of the many techniques, such as progressive muscle relaxation, that offer a way to release tension held in the body. Biofeedback therapy also provides another avenue, utilizing real-time data to help you understand and control your physiological functions. With this tool, you can learn to influence your heart rate and respiration, strengthening your capacity to return to a parasympathetic state. Adding mindfulness and meditation relieves the relentless chatter of a stressed mind. These practices encourage you to focus on each breath, each moment, fostering a sense of peace and grounding.

Incorporating these strategies into your life can transform how you experience stress, offering a path to resilience and renewal. It's about finding pockets of calm amidst the chaos, moments where the vagus nerve can guide you back to balance. Whether through deep breathing, mindful presence, biofeedback, or the gentle release of muscle tension, these techniques open the door to a new way of engaging with stress, where you're no longer at its mercy.

6.4 What about the Trauma I've Experienced?

Trauma, whether physical or emotional, leaves a profound imprint on the body, reverberating through the nervous system in ways that can disrupt our sense of equilibrium. Physical trauma, like an injury from an accident, can jolt the body into a prolonged state of vigilance as if it's bracing for the next impact. Emotional trauma, stemming from events that deeply affect us, can be equally powerful, embedding itself in the mind and body, creating patterns of tension and fear. The vagus nerve, which plays a pivotal role in regulating our stress responses, often becomes dysregulated in the wake of trauma, struggling to bring the body back to a state of calm. Instead of guiding the body towards recovery, the nerve can get stuck in a hyper-alert or shut-down cycle, making it difficult to heal and move forward.

Balancing the vagus nerve can be a cornerstone in trauma recovery, offering pathways back to safety and resilience. Working with a counselor or therapist skilled in many techniques is essential to finding the best therapies that work for you; Eye Movement Desensitization and Reprocessing (EMDR) or Polyvagal Theory can be transformative in trauma care. EMDR, for instance, helps the brain reprocess traumatic memories, reducing their emotional charge and allowing the nervous system to find a sense of peace. The Polyvagal Theory, on the other hand, emphasizes the importance of feeling safe in social contexts, using co-regulation—the calming presence of another person—to soothe the nervous system. Engaging in somatic and vagal tone balance exercises, such as those found in yoga or tai chi, encourages the body to release stored tension, fostering a sense of being grounded and safe.

Current research is shedding light on the effectiveness of vagus nerve rebalancing in trauma care. Studies have shown that stimulating the vagus nerve can reduce symptoms of post-traumatic stress disorder (PTSD), promoting a return to normalcy in daily life. Techniques like deep breathing and gentle physical activities have enhanced vagal tone, supporting the body's natural ability to recover from trauma. These practices, by promoting a state of calm and safety, help reduce the physiological arousal that keeps trauma alive in the body. Through consistent practice, individuals can retrain their nervous systems, shifting from survival mode to a place of peace and resilience.

Consider the story of Annie, a woman who endured a traumatic event that left her feeling trapped in her own body, plagued by anxiety and hyper-vigilance. With the guidance of a therapist, she began incorporating vagus nerve exercises into her daily routine. Over time, she noticed a change. The tightness in her chest eased, her sleep improved, and the world seemed less daunting. She found hope where there had been despair, discovering that the body's capacity to heal was more remarkable than she had ever imagined. Annie's experience is a testament to the potential for recovery and the power of vagus nerve rebalancing in healing from trauma.

6.5 Depression and the Vagus Nerve: Pathways to Recovery

Depression can often trace its roots back to the elusive dance of neurotransmitters and the body's stress response systems; it is a complex and pervasive condition affecting millions worldwide. At the center of this dance lies the vagus nerve, a vital player in maintaining emotional equilibrium. As we have continued to talk about, when the vagal tone is impaired, the body's ability to regulate mood and emotion suffers. This impaired vagal tone can lead to an imbalance of neurotransmitters, such as serotonin and dopamine, which are essential for stabilizing mood. A low vagal tone can lead to a cascade of depressive symptoms, leaving you trapped in a cycle of despair and fatigue. The vagus nerve's influence on the gut-brain axis also means that its dysfunction can affect gut health, further exacerbating depressive symptoms. Addressing these imbalances through targeted interventions can open new pathways to recovery.

One such intervention is vagus nerve stimulation (VNS), a complementary therapy that offers hope for those battling depression. VNS, combined with various techniques such as low-intensity exercise routines and deep breathing exercises, particularly those focused on exhalation, can stimulate the vagus nerve, enhancing its tone and promoting a calming effect. These practices encourage the body to engage the parasympathetic nervous system, fostering a sense of relaxation and reducing the grip of depression.

Research supports the potential benefits of VNS, showing that it can significantly improve mood and emotional regulation. By incorporating these exercises into their daily routines, individuals can experience a gradual lifting of depressive symptoms, much like the clouds parting to reveal the sun.

Integrating vagus nerve practices with traditional treatments can enhance their effectiveness, creating a holistic approach to depression management. Combining VNS with cognitive behavioral therapy (CBT) can help individuals reframe negative thought patterns, while pharmacological treatments address neurotransmitter imbalances. This multidimensional approach acknowledges the complexity of depression, addressing both its physiological and psychological aspects. By adopting a holistic approach, individuals can harness the body's innate healing potential, promoting resilience and emotional well-being.

Consider the story of Michael, who found himself engulfed in a deep depression following the loss of his job. Traditional treatments provided some relief, but it wasn't until he added vagus nerve exercises to his routine that he experienced a profound shift. Incorporating deep breathing exercises and gentle yoga, he noticed a gradual improvement in his mood. Over time, the darkness lifted, and he found himself engaging with life once more. Michael's journey is a testament to the power of integrating vagus nerve practices with conventional therapies, highlighting the potential for recovery and resilience in the face of depression.

6.6 Mood Stabilization: Real-Life Stories of Vagus Nerve Success

Mood stabilization is the process of achieving a steady emotional state, where fluctuations in mood are minimized, thereby allowing for consistent mental and emotional well-being. It is about finding that equilibrium where external circumstances do not dictate your mood, but instead, you remain grounded and resilient. The vagus nerve plays a crucial role in this balance as it is deeply involved in regulating the autonomic nervous system.

Engaging your vagus nerve can influence your body's ability to manage stress and maintain emotional well-being. Consistent engagement of the vagus nerve strengthens its tone, which enhances its ability to regulate emotions and respond adaptively to stressors.

Balancing the autonomic nervous system through vagus nerve engagement involves physiological processes that stabilize mood. When you consistently practice techniques that stimulate the vagus nerve, such as deep breathing exercises or cold exposure, you enhance its tone. Stimulating the vagus nerve then promotes a calm and balanced state, reducing the likelihood of emotional turbulence. The benefits of such engagement are far-reaching, providing a foundation for emotional resilience and stability. It fosters a sense of inner peace and empowers you to navigate life's challenges with a steady heart.

Real-life examples illustrate the transformative power of these practices. Consider James, a busy professional whose life was a whirlwind of deadlines and stress. He found a profound sense of balance by dedicating ten minutes daily to mindful breathing and progressive relaxation. His colleagues noted his newfound calm, and James felt more centered and less reactive, even in high-pressure situations. Then there's Maria, a mother juggling the demands of family and work. She incorporated gentle yoga and humming into her routine, which not only helped her manage stress but also improved her interactions with her children. These stories highlight the effectiveness of vagus nerve practices in achieving mood stabilization and enhancing quality of life.

Community and support play a significant role in maintaining this stability. Engaging with others who share similar goals can provide motivation and hold you accountable. Building a support network for emotional health, such as joining a group focused on mindfulness or attending community workshops, can offer valuable shared experiences. These connections create a sense of belonging and reinforce positive habits, making mood stabilization more attainable. The power of community lies in the encouragement and understanding it provides, which bolsters individual efforts and promotes long-term success.

Experts agree on the long-term benefits of mood stabilization through the engagement of the vagus nerve. Mental health professionals emphasize that consistent practice can lead to lasting emotional stability, reducing the impact of stress and enhancing overall well-being. Research supports these claims, showing that individuals who regularly engage in these practices experience improved mental health outcomes and greater resilience. This expert analysis underscores the potential of vagus nerve engagement as a tool for achieving and maintaining emotional balance, offering a pathway to a more stable and fulfilling life.

As we conclude this chapter, it's clear that the vagus nerve holds the key to emotional well-being, offering practical solutions for mood stabilization. The path to balance involves consistent practice and engagement, supported by community and expert guidance. Understanding these principles sets the stage for the next chapter, where we will continue to explore the vagus nerve's transformative potential in enhancing overall health and vitality when confronted with pain and inflammation.

Chapter 7: Pain, Inflammation, and the Vagus Nerve

Take a moment to imagine your body as a finely tuned orchestra, where each instrument represents an aspect of your health. When everything is in harmony, you feel vibrant and balanced. But when pain strikes, it's as if you are suddenly out of tune and playing a totally different song that the rest of the orchestra. We continue to discuss this, but it bears repeating- at the heart of this intricate ensemble lies the vagus nerve, a conductor of sorts, quietly guiding the body's perception and modulation of pain. This nerve does more than send signals; it orchestrates a complex interplay between the brain and body, influencing how we experience and respond to pain.

7.1 Pain Perception

The vagus nerve's influence on pain perception is profound, stemming from its role in regulating neurotransmitters and interacting with the limbic system. The limbic system is a network of interconnected brain structures that is crucial in regulating emotions, memory, motivation, and behavior. Neurotransmitters such as endorphins and serotonin, often referred to as the body's natural painkillers, play a pivotal role in this process. They work by modulating the intensity of pain signals, much like a dimmer switch adjusts the light in a room. Endorphins, for instance, bind to opioid receptors in the brain, reducing pain perception and inducing a sense of well-being. Opioid receptors are a family of protein receptors found in the central nervous system (CNS) and other tissues. They are crucial in pain perception, reward, euphoria, and other physiological functions. Conversely, serotonin plays a critical role in mood regulation and pain inhibition, ensuring pain signals do not overwhelm the nervous system. The vagus nerve's activity directly influences the production and release of these neurotransmitters, highlighting its central role in maintaining pain balance.

Moreover, the vagus nerve's connection to the limbic system further underscores its impact on pain perception. Specifically, the limbic system is responsible for processing emotions and memories, and its interaction with the vagus nerve can influence how we perceive and interpret pain. When the vagus nerve functions optimally, it helps regulate emotional responses to pain, reducing the sensation of discomfort and promoting a calm state. This connection explains why emotional stress can exacerbate physical pain, as an overactive limbic system can heighten pain perception. The vagus nerve acts as a buffer by modulating limbic activity, helping to regulate pain and promote a more balanced emotional state.

The mechanisms through which vagus nerve stimulation (VNS) alleviates pain are intricate and fascinating. By altering neural pathways, VNS can inhibit pain signals before they reach conscious awareness, like a traffic controller rerouting cars to prevent congestion. This process involves modulating pain pathways in the brainstem and spinal cord, where the vagus nerve exerts its influence. By enhancing the pain threshold, VNS effectively raises the bar for what is perceived as painful, allowing individuals to tolerate discomfort more easily. Clinical trials have shown that both invasive and noninvasive VNS devices can significantly reduce pain in conditions like fibromyalgia, abdominal pain, and headaches, offering hope to those seeking relief from chronic pain.

Scientific studies continue to validate the efficacy of VNS in pain management. Research has demonstrated that VNS not only alleviates pain but also enhances overall well-being by promoting the release of endorphins and serotonin. These findings underscore the potential of VNS as a therapeutic tool, providing a non-pharmacological option for managing chronic pain. The ability of VNS to modulate pain pathways and enhance neurotransmitter activity represents a promising avenue for those grappling with persistent pain.

Several techniques can be easily incorporated into daily life for those seeking practical ways to harness the vagus nerve's pain-relieving potential. Tapping or EFT (Emotional Freedom Technique) and acupressure, for instance, are simple yet effective methods for stimulating the vagus nerve. By applying gentle pressure to specific points on the body, these techniques activate the nerves and promote relaxation. Similarly, gentle stretching exercises like yoga and tai chi can enhance vagal tone, reduce muscle tension, and alleviate pain. These practices encourage the body to enter a state of rest and recovery, fostering a sense of ease and comfort.

Reflection: Exploring Pain Relief

Consider taking a moment to reflect on your personal experiences with pain.

How does your body react when you encounter discomfort?

Are there specific techniques that have helped you manage pain in the past?

Jot down your observations and consider exploring new practices that activate the vagus nerve, such as tapping or gentle stretching. By experimenting with these techniques, you can discover what works best for your body and empower yourself to take control of your pain management journey.

Remember that consistency is key as you explore these vagus nerve activation methods. Regular practice can enhance vagal tone over time, building resilience and reducing the impact of pain on your daily life. With patience and persistence, you can develop a deeper connection with your body, fostering a sense of well-being that extends beyond pain relief.

7.2 Reducing Inflammation Through Vagal Stimulation

Inflammation is the body's natural response to injury or infection, like an alert system that calls upon immune cells to heal and protect. While acute inflammation is beneficial, chronic inflammation can become a relentless storm, wreaking havoc on your health. Here, the vagus nerve emerges as a crucial ally. It acts like a wise mediator, calming the inflammatory response and preventing it from spiraling out of control. The nerve interacts closely with the immune system, regulating the production of cytokines—proteins that act as messengers in inflammation. Think of cytokines as traffic signals that can direct the immune system's flow smoothly or cause gridlock and chaos. When the vagus nerve is stimulated, it helps maintain a balanced cytokine production, reducing unnecessary inflammation and promoting healing.

Stimulation of the vagus nerve has also shown impressive anti-inflammatory effects, shifting the immune system from a heightened state of alertness to a more controlled and calmer stance. It's like turning down the volume on an overzealous alarm. This process involves decreasing the levels of pro-inflammatory cytokines, often elevated in chronic conditions, while simultaneously enhancing pathways that promote healing. This dual action helps mitigate inflammation and supports the body's overall resilience. By engaging the vagus nerve, you can guide your immune system to respond more intelligently, reducing inflammation while preserving its ability to combat real threats.

Specific inflammatory conditions have demonstrated marked improvement through vagal stimulation. Rheumatoid arthritis, a painful condition in which the immune system mistakenly attacks the joints, has shown relief with vagal modulation. Inflammatory bowel disease, characterized by chronic digestive tract inflammation, also benefits from the calming effects of the vagus nerve. Chronic fatigue syndrome, often accompanied by inflammation and debilitating exhaustion, shows potential for improvement as well. These examples underscore the broad applicability of vagal stimulation in managing inflammation-related diseases, offering hope for those seeking relief from persistent symptoms.

Lifestyle changes can significantly enhance vagal tone and combat inflammation, providing a foundation for improved health. Incorporating anti-inflammatory foods into your diet is one step. Foods rich in omega-3 fatty acids can reduce inflammation. These foods include salmon, tuna, a variety of nuts and seeds, which can help reduce inflammation. Leafy greens, such as spinach and kale, are also beneficial. Stress management techniques play a pivotal role, as chronic stress can exacerbate inflammation. Practices such as mindfulness meditation, deep breathing exercises, and yoga help soothe the mind and stimulate the vagus nerve, promoting an anti-inflammatory response. By making these conscious adjustments, you create a supportive environment for your body, enhancing its natural ability to heal and reducing the burden of inflammation.

Incorporating these habits into your daily life can be transformative. Imagine starting your day with a bowl gluten-free grains, such as millet, amaranth, sorghum or buckwheat, topped with berries, cherries, hemp hearts, flax seeds, and walnuts, followed by a brief morning yoga session. Pause, breathe deeply, and ground yourself throughout the day, especially during stressful situations. As you nourish your body with wholesome foods and practice mindfulness, you'll likely notice a shift in inflammation and your overall sense of well-being. These small, consistent steps can profoundly impact your health, supporting the vagus nerve in its role as a guardian of balance and healing.

7.3 Alternative Pain Relief Techniques

In the pursuit of pain relief, many people turn to complementary therapies that align with the body's natural healing processes. One such practice is acupuncture, an ancient modality rooted in Traditional Chinese Medicine. By inserting fine needles into specific acupoints along energy pathways throughout the body called meridians, acupuncture aims to balance the flow of Qi (life energy). This technique not only promotes deep relaxation but also positively influences vagal tone. Research suggests that acupuncture can stimulate vagal activity, enhancing the nervous system's ability to regulate pain. As the needles engage acupoints, they activate the vagus nerve, helping to calm the body and mind.

Herbal medicine, used for centuries to address pain and inflammation, provides natural alternatives to conventional drugs. Some of the most effective herbs include:

- **Turmeric (Curcuma longa)** – Contains **curcumin**, a potent anti-inflammatory that helps reduce joint pain and stiffness, particularly in arthritis.

- **Ginger (Zingiber officinale)** – Works similarly to NSAIDs by inhibiting the production of **prostaglandins**, hormone-like compounds that play key roles in pain, inflammation, and fever.

- **Boswellia (Boswellia serrata)** – Also known as Indian frankincense, contains **boswellic acids** that block inflammatory pathways, making it effective for chronic conditions like osteoarthritis and rheumatoid arthritis.

- **Willow bark (Salix alba)** – Often referred to as "nature's aspirin," it contains **salicin**, which the body converts into **salicylic acid**, offering pain relief with fewer gastrointestinal side effects than synthetic aspirin.

- **Devil's claw (Harpagophytum procumbens)** – Widely used for musculoskeletal pain, including lower back pain, osteoarthritis, and tendonitis.

- **Capsaicin** – Derived from chili peppers, it helps relieve nerve and joint pain by depleting **substance P**, a neuropeptide involved in pain signaling.

- **CBD (cannabidiol)** – A compound from hemp that interacts with the **endocannabinoid system (ECS)**—a regulatory network involved in pain perception, mood, sleep, appetite, memory, immunity, and cardiovascular health.

Incorporating these herbs into a holistic pain management plan can offer effective relief with fewer side effects than pharmaceutical drugs.

Essential oils, with their alluring fragrance, provide additional support in pain management. Oils such as lavender and chamomile are widely known for their soothing properties and ability to promote relaxation. When inhaled or applied topically, these oils can stimulate the olfactory system, which influences the limbic system—the brain's emotional center. (Check to see if your essential oils are suitable for topical application; they may need to be mixed with a carrier oil). This interaction encourages the release of endorphins, the body's natural pain relievers, and enhances vagal tone. Incorporating essential oils into your routine can be as simple as adding a few drops to a warm bath or using a diffuser to fill your space with calming aromas. This sensory experience not only aids in relaxation but also complements the effects of vagus nerve stimulation, creating a multi-faceted approach to pain relief.

Integrating these holistic therapies and others with vagus nerve practices can lead to a complementary pain management plan tailored to your unique needs. I will discuss these holistic therapies in greater detail in my next book, "*My Holistic Vagus Nerve Toolkit: A Naturopathic Doctor's Strategies to Promote a Balanced Nervous System for Digestive Health, Pain Relief, Mental Health, and Decresed Inflammation*".

Begin by identifying the practices that resonate with you, whether acupuncture, aromatherapy, or a combination of these techniques. Consider the timing of these practices, as incorporating them into your daily routine can maximize their benefits. For instance, schedule an acupuncture session in the evening to unwind after a long day, followed by a relaxing bath infused with essential oils. This intentional approach allows you to harness the synergistic effects of multiple modalities, enhancing overall pain reduction and improving your quality of life.

The benefits of a multimodal approach extend beyond physical relief, profoundly impacting emotional well-being. By combining various therapies, you create a comprehensive support system that addresses pain's physical and emotional aspects. This approach not only alleviates discomfort but also fosters a sense of empowerment and resilience. As you explore these complementary techniques, please note how they influence your pain levels, mood, and overall sense of balance. This awareness can guide you in refining your pain management plan, ensuring it evolves alongside your needs.

Testimonials from individuals who have embraced alternative pain relief techniques highlight the transformative power of a holistic approach. Consider Tiffany, who struggled with chronic back pain for years. After incorporating acupuncture and aromatherapy into her routine, she experienced a significant reduction in pain and an enhanced sense of well-being. "Living pain-free with a holistic approach has given me a new lease on life," she shares. Similarly, Mike found relief from migraines through a combination of acupuncture and essential oils. "Finding relief through combined therapies has been a game-changer for me. It's not just about the physical pain; it's about feeling whole again," he explains. These stories underscore the potential of complementary therapies to manage pain and enrich your quality of life.

7.4 Case Studies in Chronic Pain Management

Emily's story offers a glimpse into the life-altering potential of vagus nerve stimulation for managing fibromyalgia, a condition that had long dictated her daily life. Her days were filled with persistent pain, fatigue, and the constant challenge of maintaining a semblance of normalcy. Traditional treatments provided little relief, prompting Emily to seek alternatives. She found a path forward only when she discovered the potential of vagal stimulation. Emily began incorporating tailored vagal stimulation routines into her daily regimen, focusing on gentle exercises and mindfulness practices that engaged her parasympathetic nervous system. Over time, she noticed a gradual decrease in pain and increased energy levels. This transformation wasn't a miracle cure but rather a testament to the power of consistency and adaptation.

Similarly, John's battle with persistent back pain showcases the diverse applications of vagus nerve techniques. Years of discomfort had taken their toll, affecting not only his physical health but also his mental and emotional well-being. After learning about vagus nerve stimulation, John decided to explore its potential. He incorporated specific lifestyle modifications to support his vagal tone, including prioritizing a balanced diet rich in anti-inflammatory foods and engaging in daily breathing exercises. The results were gradual but profound. As John's vagal tone improved, he experienced a decrease in pain intensity and an enhanced ability to manage stress. This newfound relief allowed him to regain a sense of control over his life, free from the constant shadow of pain.

These case studies highlight the diversity of conditions and outcomes associated with targeted vagus nerve practices. Beyond fibromyalgia and back pain, similar successes have been observed in arthritis management, where individuals have reported reduced joint inflammation and improved mobility. Neuropathic pain, often characterized by burning and tingling sensations, has also shown responsiveness to vagal stimulation, offering hope to those seeking relief from this challenging condition. Each of these stories is a testament to the potential of vagus nerve techniques in transforming chronic pain management.

The strategies and techniques employed in each case vary but share common elements of personalization and commitment. Tailored vagal stimulation routines are designed to address the unique needs of the individual, taking into account specific pain triggers and lifestyle factors. For Emily, this meant incorporating mindfulness practices that calmed her mind and body, while for John, it involved dietary changes and focused breathing exercises. These personalized approaches emphasize the importance of consistency and adaptation, enabling individuals to develop resilience and gradually enhance their quality of life. They found a renewed sense of hope and empowerment by embracing these practices.

Lessons from these case studies offer valuable insights for anyone navigating the complexities of chronic pain management. Consistency emerges as a key factor in achieving positive outcomes, as regular engagement with vagus nerve practices reinforces their benefits over time. Adaptation is equally essential, as everyone's journey is unique, requiring adjustments to find the right balance. Personalization is crucial, enabling individuals to tailor their pain relief practices to suit their needs and preferences. This approach empowers individuals to actively participate in their health, fostering a sense of ownership and control.

Applying vagus nerve techniques in chronic pain management highlights the body's innate healing abilities. Individuals can tap into a resource that alleviates pain and promotes overall well-being by engaging the vagus nerve. These case studies serve as a reminder that the path to pain relief is not one-size-fits-all but rather a dynamic process that evolves with each individual's needs. As you explore the potential of vagus nerve practices, consider how these lessons can inform your approach, guiding you toward a life of greater comfort and balance.

As we wrap up this chapter, it becomes clear that the vagus nerve is a powerful ally in managing pain and inflammation—quietly regulating your body's response, soothing discomfort, and supporting healing from within. Whether through gentle stretches, anti-inflammatory foods, or alternative therapies, these practices reveal the body's innate ability to restore balance. Yet, healing is not confined to waking hours. The vagus nerve continues its work even while you sleep, playing a vital role in your body's nightly renewal process. In the next chapter, we'll shift our focus to how this incredible nerve influences your sleep—guiding you into deeper rest, regulating your circadian rhythm, and helping you rise each day with renewed energy and clarity.

Chapter 8: Vagus Nerve and Sleep Optimization

Picture a restless night where your mind races like a carousel, each thought a brightly lit horse refusing to slow down. Sleep eludes you despite your best attempts to find rest, leaving you weary and disoriented. This frustrating cycle is all too familiar for many, and it is where the vagus nerve's role in sleep becomes a focal point of understanding and healing. The vagus nerve, an unsung hero in your body's intricate superhighway system, significantly impacts your ability to achieve restorative sleep. When functioning optimally, it helps regulate sleep cycles, ensuring that you drift smoothly into deep stages of rest. However, when imbalances arise, the harmony is disrupted, leading to a cascade of sleep disturbances that affect your well-being.

8.1 Sleep Architecture

The vagus nerve plays a crucial role in maintaining the body's sleep architecture, which describes the structure and sequence of sleep stages. It influences how you transition from light to deep sleep into REM (Rapid Eye Movement) phases, which are essential for mental and emotional rejuvenation. Poor vagal tone, often stemming from chronic stress or lifestyle factors, can impede these transitions, disrupting the delicate balance needed for quality sleep. You may struggle with insomnia, a condition characterized by persistent difficulty in falling or staying asleep. Insomnia often results from an overactive mind or elevated stress levels, both of which can strain the vagus nerve and perpetuate a cycle of sleeplessness. Sleep apnea, characterized by interrupted breathing during sleep, is also linked to vagus nerve dysfunction. Disrupted breathing patterns can trigger frequent awakenings throughout the night, depriving you of the deep, restorative sleep your body craves.

The impact of stress and anxiety on sleep is profound, creating a cyclical relationship where poor sleep exacerbates stress and vice versa. Elevated cortisol levels, a common stress hormone, can interfere with your body's natural sleep-wake cycle, making it difficult to achieve restful sleep. The vagus nerve is pivotal in mitigating these effects, acting as a calming force that helps lower elevated nighttime cortisol levels and promote relaxation. Yet, when stress overwhelms this system, the nerve's ability to regulate these hormones diminishes, leading to stress-induced insomnia. Understanding this connection is crucial, as it enables you to address the underlying causes of your sleep disturbances.

To enhance sleep quality through vagal activation, consider adopting specific strategies supporting the nerve's function, such as creating a bedtime routine that signals your body that it's time to wind down. Incorporate deep breathing exercises into this routine, focusing on slow, diaphragmatic breaths that stimulate the vagus nerve and encourage a state of calm. Weighted blankets can also promote relaxation by providing a gentle, comforting pressure that mimics the sensation of a warm embrace, helping to soothe an overactive nervous system. Dietary changes, such as consuming foods rich in magnesium and tryptophan, can support sleep by promoting melatonin production, a hormone that regulates the sleep-wake cycle.

The concept of sleep architecture underscores the importance of each sleep stage and the transitions between them. Deep sleep stages are critical for physical restoration, while REM sleep fosters cognitive processing and emotional regulation. The vagus nerve's activity influences these stages by modulating the balance of the autonomic nervous system, ensuring deep and restorative sleep. A healthy vagal tone promotes shorter sleep latency, allowing you to fall asleep more quickly and enjoy extended periods of deep sleep.

Assessing vagus nerve-related sleep disturbances requires a thoughtful approach. Sleep diaries can be invaluable for tracking patterns and identifying triggers that may disrupt sleep. By recording your sleep habits, you gain valuable insights into the factors influencing your rest, empowering you to make informed changes. Wearable sleep monitors offer another layer of insight, providing data on sleep stages, duration, and disturbances. These tools can help you pinpoint issues related to vagal dysfunction and tailor interventions to enhance sleep quality.

Interactive Element: Journal Your Sleep

Creating and utilizing a Sleep Diary can provide vital information and tremendously change your health.

Sleep Diary Template

1. ***Bedtime and Wake Time:*** *Record your bedtime and wake time daily.*
2. ***Sleep Duration:*** *Note the total hours of sleep you achieve each night.*
3. ***Sleep Quality:*** *Rate your sleep quality on a scale of 1 to 10.*
4. ***Nighttime Awakenings:*** *Note any awakenings and their duration.*
5. ***Pre-Sleep Activities:*** *List activities in the hour before bed, including screen time, snacks, or relaxation exercises.*
6. ***Stress Levels:*** *Rate your stress levels on a scale of 1 to 10 before bed.*

By understanding the vagus nerve's impact on sleep and implementing these strategies, you can cultivate a more harmonious relationship with rest, paving the way for a more balanced and rejuvenated life.

8.2 Evening Routines for Better Sleep: Vagus Nerve Activation

As the sun dips below the horizon, signaling the end of another day, the transition into evening offers a unique opportunity to prepare your mind and body for restful sleep. Crafting an intentional evening routine can significantly impact the quality of your rest by stimulating the vagus nerve, leading to a cascade of calming effects. One simple yet effective approach is incorporating warm herbal teas into your nightly routine. Chamomile and valerian teas are renowned for their soothing properties, gently lulling both mind and body into a state of relaxation. Sipping a warm beverage becomes a mindful practice, encouraging you to slow down and savor the moment.

Again, gentle stretching or restorative yoga can complement this pre-sleep routine, promoting relaxation and alleviating tension accumulated throughout the day. Restorative yoga, in particular, involves holding poses for extended periods, allowing the body to unwind fully. This practice doesn't just target the muscles; it engages the parasympathetic nervous system, fostering a sense of tranquility that prepares you for sleep. As you move through each pose, focus on your breath, allowing it to deepen and slow, stimulating the vagus nerve and reinforcing the body's relaxation response.

Anyone should not underestimate the power of sensory experiences in promoting vagal activation. Our senses can profoundly affect our state of mind, making them a valuable tool in your evening routine. You can use calming essential oils, such as lavender, which has been shown to reduce anxiety and improve sleep quality. Diffusing a few drops of essential oil in your bedroom can create an atmosphere of peace and serenity, inviting restful sleep. Pair this with soft, soothing music or nature sounds, which can lull you into a relaxed state by masking disruptive noises and encouraging a focus on the present moment. Allow these gentle melodies to wash over you, easing the transition from wakefulness to sleep.

Digital detoxing is another crucial aspect of enhancing vagal tone and preparing your body for sleep. The glow of screens emits blue light, which can interfere with melatonin production and disrupt your body's natural sleep-wake cycle. Establishing a no-device rule at least an hour before bed can help mitigate these effects, allowing your mind to unwind from the constant barrage of information. Instead of scrolling through your phone, consider engaging in reading or journaling. These activities help distract from screens and provide a space for reflection and relaxation, clearing your mind before sleep.

Optimizing your sleep environment is equally vital in supporting vagal activation. Ensure your bedroom is conducive to rest by using blackout curtains to block any intrusive light, creating a dark sanctuary that signals your body it's time for sleep. Maintaining a cool room temperature can also enhance comfort, as your body's core temperature naturally drops during sleep. A cool temperature environment supports this process, promoting more profound and restorative rest. Consistency in your sleep schedule is another cornerstone of good sleep hygiene. To help regulate your body's internal clock, start by going to bed and waking up at the same time each day, making it easier to fall asleep and wake up feeling refreshed.

Incorporating mindfulness, meditation, and breathwork into your evening routine can bolster these efforts. These practices encourage focusing on the present moment, reducing stress and anxiety that might otherwise keep you awake at night. Simple exercises like this breathing exercise can work wonders in calming the nervous system. Inhale deeply through the nose, hold it for a few seconds, and then exhale slowly through the mouth. Repeat this exercise until you relax. As you lie in bed, let your breath guide you; with each exhale, tension is released, and you draw closer to sleep.

8.3 The Role of the Vagus Nerve in Circadian Rhythm Regulation

Our bodies are guided by an internal clock known as the circadian rhythm, a 24-hour cycle that orchestrates numerous physiological processes, including the sleep-wake cycle. At the heart of this intricate system lies the suprachiasmatic nucleus (SCN) in the hypothalamus, a tiny brain region that functions as the master clock. It receives direct input from light through the eyes and cues the timing of various bodily functions, including hormone release, body temperature regulation, and sleep patterns. The SCN's ability to sync with the external environment helps maintain the rhythm that dictates when we feel alert and when we feel sleepy, aligning us with the natural day-night cycle.

The vagus nerve, a crucial player in our body's communication network, influences circadian rhythms by interacting with the SCN and other systems. The vagus nerve is intricately connected to the production and release of melatonin, a hormone that promotes sleep. When the SCN signals the onset of darkness, it triggers a cascade of events that culminate in melatonin secretion from the pineal gland. The pineal gland is a tiny, cone-shaped gland in the brain's center. It is part of the endocrine system that produces and secretes melatonin, which is how it regulates sleep-wake cycles and circadian rhythms.

The vagus nerve supports this process by ensuring the autonomic nervous system maintains balance, allowing melatonin to flow unhindered and guiding us gently into sleep. Beyond melatonin, the vagus nerve influences body temperature and metabolism, both key components of circadian regulation. During the night, your body temperature naturally falls, signaling the time for rest. The vagus nerve plays a partial role in orchestrating this drop, which helps modulate thermoregulatory processes. Similarly, metabolism slows during sleep, conserving energy and allowing for restoration and repair. The vagus nerve maintains these physiological changes and supports a seamless transition into and through the night.

Consider incorporating practices that engage the vagus nerve to align your circadian rhythms and enhance sleep quality. Exposure to natural light during the day can help calibrate your internal clock. Morning sunlight, in particular, strengthens the signals sent to the SCN, reinforcing the rhythm that dictates when to wake and sleep. Regular exposure to daylight encourages the release of serotonin, a precursor to melatonin, setting the stage for restful nights. Consuming meals at consistent intervals further supports circadian alignment. Eating regularly helps synchronize the body's clocks, reinforcing the cues guiding your sleep-wake cycle. This routine also aids digestion and energy regulation, improving overall health and well-being.

Recent research has shown the connection between the vagus nerve and the synchronization of the circadian rhythm. Studies have demonstrated that light therapy, commonly used to treat seasonal affective disorder (SAD) and other circadian rhythm-related disturbances, can enhance vagal tone. Increasing exposure to bright light during the day can stimulate the vagus nerve, leading to improved sleep and better mood regulation. Chronobiology research continues to unravel the complex relationship between circadian rhythms and the vagus nerve. Findings suggest that consistent engagement of the vagus nerve through lifestyle practices can enhance the body's ability to adapt to environmental changes, thereby fostering resilience against disruptions such as jet lag or shift work.

The connection between the vagus nerve and circadian rhythms provides a pathway to enhanced sleep and overall well-being. Understanding and nurturing this relationship can create a harmonious balance between your body's internal clock and the external world. Engaging the vagus nerve through intentional practices supports restorative sleep and enhances your capacity to thrive in a world that often challenges your natural rhythms. As you explore these strategies, remember that small, consistent changes can lead to profound improvements in your sleep and well-being.

8.4 Case Studies: Success Stories in Sleep Improvement

In the quiet hours of the night, when most of the world is at rest, some find themselves caught in a cycle of wakefulness and fatigue. This cycle was the reality for Holly, a dedicated night-shift nurse who struggled with the demands of her irregular schedule. Her sleep was fragmented, leaving her feeling perpetually drained. By incorporating vagus nerve techniques, Holly transformed her sleep patterns dramatically. She began by adopting a consistent pre-sleep ritual tailored to her unique schedule. Holly committed to a wind-down routine that included dimming the lights and practicing deep breathing exercises designed to activate her vagus nerve. This simple yet effective practice helped signal to her body that it was time to relax, even when her external environment suggested otherwise. Within weeks, Holly noticed a marked improvement in her ability to fall asleep quickly and stay asleep longer. These changes rejuvenated her energy levels and enhanced her performance during demanding night shifts.

Mark, a retiree in his seventies, battled with frequent awakenings throughout the night in another corner of the world. His sleep was shallow, often interrupted by bouts of restlessness that left him weary each morning. Determined to reclaim restful sleep, Mark explored vagus nerve activation as a potential remedy. He integrated gentle breathing techniques into his nightly routine, focusing on long, slow breaths that encouraged relaxation. Mark also embraced guided relaxation tapes, which combined calming music with soothing narratives, further promoting vagal activation. Over time, these techniques reduced his sleep fragmentation, allowing him to experience longer periods of uninterrupted rest. As a result, Mark enjoyed increased daytime alertness and an improved mood, feeling more vibrant and engaged with life.

The long-term benefits observed in these stories extend beyond the realm of sleep. Holly and Mark experienced enhanced cognitive function, with greater clarity and focus throughout the day. This improvement in mental acuity was accompanied by a noticeable uplift in their overall mood, underscoring the profound impact of restorative sleep on emotional well-being. These interventions' sustained benefits highlight the vagus nerve's power in fostering holistic health, demonstrating that small, intentional changes can yield significant rewards.

Sleep specialists have weighed in on the effectiveness of these approaches, offering insights into the broader applications of vagus nerve interventions. Dr. Sarah Evans, a renowned sleep researcher, highlights the crucial role of the vagus nerve in regulating sleep. She notes that by engaging this nerve through targeted techniques, individuals can tap into the body's natural relaxation responses, paving the way for improved sleep quality. Dr. Evans advocates for integrating these practices into sleep management protocols, suggesting that they offer a valuable complement to existing therapies. Her analysis underscores the potential for vagus nerve activation to become a cornerstone of sleep health, accessible to anyone willing to explore its benefits.

Professional analyses of these case studies highlight a promising area for improving sleep. Experts recommend a broader application of vagus nerve techniques, encouraging individuals to experiment with different strategies to find what resonates with their unique needs. These recommendations offer hope to many who struggle with sleep disturbances, illustrating that meaningful change is within reach through the gentle power of the vagus nerve. As you contemplate these stories, consider how these insights might inspire your path to restful sleep.

As we conclude our exploration of sleep and the vagus nerve, remember the potential of this vital connection in achieving restful nights and revitalized days. The stories shared here remind us that with the right tools and guidance, sleep can transform from a source of frustration into one of restoration. In the next chapter, we'll delve into how the vagus nerve influences digestive health, unveiling its integral role in holistic well-being.

Chapter 9: Your Digestive Health and the Vagus Nerve

Now, take a moment to visualize your digestive system as a bustling metropolis full of activity and life. The roads of this city are your intestines, where nutrients are transported and absorbed, ensuring your body has the energy it needs to thrive. But what happens when a traffic jam occurs? A traffic jam in this context is like a disruption in the gut-brain axis, a sophisticated communication network that depends heavily on the vagus nerve. This nerve acts as a superhighway, bridging the gut and the brain and facilitating a constant exchange of information critical for maintaining harmony within the body. The vagus nerve's role in digestion is profound. It regulates essential functions, including gut motility, gastric acid secretion, and nutrient absorption. When it functions optimally, it ensures your digestive system runs smoothly, like a well-designed transit system.

9.1 The Vagus Nerve and Digestion

One of the most intriguing aspects of the vagus nerve's role in digestion is its influence on cortisol, a hormone often associated with stress. Elevated cortisol levels can wreak havoc on your gut health, exacerbating inflammation and disrupting the delicate balance of your gut microbiota, commonly called "gut bugs." This imbalance can lead to a host of gastrointestinal issues, ranging from bloating to irritable bowel syndrome (IBS). In essence, the vagus nerve acts as a mediator, helping to manage stress responses and mitigate their impact on your digestive health. Promoting the "rest and digest" state encourages the production of digestive enzymes and the movement of food through your gastrointestinal tract, ensuring you get the most out of every meal.

The gut-brain axis is a marvel of biological engineering, representing the bidirectional communication between the central nervous system and the enteric nervous system, often called the "second brain." This axis is not just a conduit for physical processes; it also plays a pivotal role in your emotional and cognitive well-being. The vagus nerve is the main line of communication within this axis, transmitting sensory information from the gut to the brain and vice versa. It's fascinating to note that approximately 80-90% of the vagus nerve's fibers are afferent, meaning they carry signals from the gut to the brain. This gut-to-brain highway highlights the gut's profound impact on mental health, with studies suggesting that a balanced gut can contribute to improved mood and cognitive function.

The gut microbiota, a diverse community of microorganisms living in your intestines, is integral to the gut-brain axis. These microbes are crucial in producing neurotransmitters like serotonin, often called the "happiness hormone." Interestingly, the gut produces about 90% - 95% of the body's serotonin, underscoring its influence on mood and behavior. The vagus nerve serves as a conduit for these signals, allowing the brain to respond to changes in the gut environment. This connection is vital for maintaining emotional balance and cognitive health, illustrating the profound impact of gut health on the mind.

Supporting the vagus nerve and digestion through diet is crucial for maintaining this intricate balance. Mindful eating is a practice that encourages you to savor each bite, fostering a deeper connection with your body's hunger and satiety cues. This awareness can enhance digestion and promote a sense of satisfaction and well-being. Incorporating fermented foods and probiotic-rich options, such as yogurt or sauerkraut, into your diet can support a healthy gut microbiota, bolstering the gut-brain connection. Probiotics, beneficial bacteria in these foods, help maintain a balanced microbiome, which can positively influence vagal activity and digestion. As you navigate your dietary choices, consider the profound impact they have not only on your physical health but also on your mental and emotional well-being. As a key player in the gut-brain axis, the vagus nerve reminds us of the interconnectedness of our body's systems and the potential for holistic healing through mindful nourishment.

Interactive Element: Mindful Eating Exercise

Set aside a quiet moment for your next meal. Begin by taking a deep breath, allowing yourself to be fully present in the moment. As you eat, focus on each bite's flavors, textures, and aromas. Chew slowly, savoring each mouthful, and notice how your body responds. Are you feeling more satisfied? More connected to your meal? This exercise promotes a deeper awareness of your body's signals. It can help cultivate a more mindful approach to eating, supporting your digestive health and the function of your vagus nerve.

9.2 Vagal Influence and Digestion Issues

Picture a time when you ate your favorite meal, only to feel uncomfortably full and nauseous hours later. This lingering discomfort may be linked to gastroparesis, where the vagus nerve cannot effectively stimulate the stomach muscles. When this nerve fails to function correctly, food remains in the stomach longer than it should, resulting in symptoms such as chronic nausea, early satiety, and even vomiting of undigested food. The upper abdominal discomfort accompanying these symptoms can be distressing, both physically and emotionally, as it disrupts your ability to enjoy meals and social gatherings. The vagus nerve ensures that the stomach empties at the right pace, coordinating with digestive enzymes to break down food effectively.

Imagine experiencing persistent indigestion, as if a stone sat in your stomach. This sensation is often linked to dyspepsia, where the vagus nerve's regulation of gastric acid secretion becomes imbalanced. The result? The stomach struggles to produce adequate acids or enzymes necessary for proper digestion. Symptoms like belching, a poor appetite, and generalized upper gastrointestinal discomfort can manifest, leaving you feeling bloated and uneasy. It's as if your digestive system is working in overdrive without the proper support, leading to inefficiency and irritation. When functioning optimally, the vagus nerve ensures that gastric juices are secreted in the right amounts, facilitating the breakdown of food and preventing such discomfort.

Consider the discomfort of acid reflux, where a burning sensation in your chest disrupts your day. This experience, often linked to gastroesophageal reflux disease (GERD), can be aggravated by impaired vagal signaling. The lower esophageal sphincter—a valve between the esophagus and stomach—relies on proper vagal function to maintain its tone. When it fails to tighten properly, stomach acid can flow back into the esophagus, causing heartburn, regurgitation of sour liquid, and even chest discomfort. Chronic cough and hoarseness may occur if the acid reaches the larynx. These symptoms are not just physical; they can significantly impact your quality of life, leading to disrupted sleep and a reduced enjoyment of certain foods.

Swallowing difficulties, or dysphagia, can be unsettling. Imagine the sensation of food sticking in your throat or struggling to swallow. This issue arises when the coordinated contraction of muscles in the throat and esophagus, partially reliant on vagal innervation, becomes disrupted. The resulting uncoordinated or weak contractions can lead to coughing, choking during meals, or the need for liquid to wash down food. Such experiences can turn the simple act of eating into a source of anxiety, affecting social interactions and nutritional intake. The vagus nerve plays a vital role in ensuring that these muscles function harmoniously, enabling food to be moved from the mouth to the stomach.

Think of your small intestine as a moving sidewalk, similar to those found in airports, which moves food along to be digested and absorbed. When the vagus nerve's regulation of peristalsis—the wave-like contractions in the intestines—is impaired, small intestinal dysmotility can result. This dysfunction results in slower or uncoordinated movement of food, leading to bloating, excess gas, and abdominal cramping. If left unchecked, it can lead to bacterial overgrowth and malabsorption, resulting in nutrient deficiencies. The vagus nerve ensures that food moves efficiently through the digestive tract, allowing optimal nutrient absorption and preventing such issues.

Constipation or irregular bowel movements are often linked to a sluggish digestive system. Although its role here is supportive, the vagus nerve helps regulate colon motility, especially in the first half or so of the colon. When the vagal tone is underactive, transit time slows, resulting in infrequent bowel movements and a sensation of incomplete bowel movements. Straining during bowel movements and passing hard or lumpy stools can result from this imbalance, impacting your daily comfort and health. The vagus nerve's influence on the colon is subtle yet significant, maintaining regularity and ease in bowel movements.

Imagine the discomfort of persistent bloating, where your abdomen feels distended and full. This functional bloating can occur when there's a mismatch between gastrointestinal distension and sensory feedback to the brain. The body perceives normal amounts of gas or fluid as excessively uncomfortable, leading to feelings of pressure and fullness. The vagus nerve modulates this sensory feedback, helping the brain accurately interpret signals from the gut. Even small amounts of gas can cause significant discomfort when this function is impaired, impacting your overall well-being and confidence.

9.3 Managing IBS and Other Digestive Issues with Vagus Techniques

Irritable Bowel Syndrome (IBS) is often a frustrating and perplexing condition characterized by symptoms like abdominal pain, bloating, and irregular bowel movements. Understanding the connection between IBS and the vagus nerve can shed light on how this nerve's imbalances contribute to such symptoms, offering a pathway to relief. The vagus nerve plays a pivotal role in regulating the sensitivity of the gut and its response to stimuli.

When the vagal tone is compromised, the gut can become hypersensitive, overreacting to normal digestive processes. This heightened sensitivity can manifest as the hallmark symptoms of IBS, where the gut's response to food and stress is amplified, leading to discomfort and disruption in daily life.

Chronic stress is a notorious exacerbator of IBS symptoms, acting as a catalyst that intensifies the gut's response. When you're stressed, the body's fight-or-flight response kicks in, often sidelining the rest-and-digest functions governed by the vagus nerve. This shift can lead to alterations in gut motility, causing either diarrhea or constipation, which are hallmark symptoms of IBS. The connection between stress and IBS highlights the importance of managing stress levels to maintain a healthy gut. Techniques that engage the vagus nerve, such as deep breathing, meditation, or gentle yoga, can help mitigate stress's impact, promoting a calm state that supports digestive health.

The vagus nerve's influence on gut sensitivity is significant. It acts like a regulator, ensuring the gut's response to stimuli remains balanced. When the vagal tone is optimal, the gut processes food smoothly, with minimal discomfort. But when this tone is impaired, the gut's sensitivity can spiral out of control, leading to the pain and irregularity associated with IBS. Enhancing vagal function can help recalibrate the gut's responses, reducing symptoms and improving overall digestive health. Engaging in practices that stimulate the vagus nerve can restore this balance, offering a noninvasive approach to managing IBS.

Addressing IBS symptoms through vagus nerve techniques requires a holistic approach. It's about creating a lifestyle that supports vagal tone and reduces stress. This lifestyle might include incorporating regular physical activity that you enjoy, as exercise can boost vagal function and improve mood. A supportive social network can enhance emotional well-being, indirectly benefiting digestive health. Engaging in mindful and nutrient-rich eating practices, where you pay attention to your body's hunger cues and savor each bite, can also support vagal function and digestion.

By taking these steps, you can create an environment where your gut feels supported and balanced.

Understanding the connection between IBS and vagal dysfunction empowers you to take control of your digestive health. It's about recognizing the role that stressors and vagal tone play in your symptoms and using this knowledge to make informed choices. Incorporating vagus nerve techniques into your daily routine can help alleviate IBS symptoms and enhance your overall quality of life. The journey to managing IBS is personal, and while it may require some trial and error, the potential benefits of enhanced vagal function are well worth the effort. As you explore these techniques, remember that you're not alone-many have found relief through similar practices, and you, too, can discover a path to better digestive health.

9.4 Dietary Tips to Support Vagus Nerve Function

When supporting the vagus nerve and overall digestive health, the foods you choose can play a pivotal role. Imagine your diet as a garden, where each choice you make plants a seed for wellness. Emphasizing anti-inflammatory foods can be a powerful strategy in this garden. These foods help reduce inflammation that can disrupt vagal function and digestion. Think of colorful berries, rich in antioxidants, or fatty fish like salmon, packed with omega-3s, as key players in this anti-inflammatory team. Omega-3s, also found in flaxseeds, are known for their ability to support brain health and reduce inflammation, making them a valuable addition to your diet. Incorporating fermented foods, such as yogurt and sauerkraut, can also enhance vagal health. These foods are rich in probiotics, the beneficial bacteria that support a healthy gut microbiome. In my next book, I'll discuss the Vagus Support Diet in detail, but the components are included below. Remember, a diverse and balanced microbiome can positively influence vagus nerve activity, promoting a harmonious gut-brain connection.

Leafy greens and cruciferous vegetables are another essential component of a vagus-friendly diet. These vegetables, which include kale, spinach, broccoli, and Brussels sprouts, are nutrient powerhouses. They provide essential vitamins and minerals that support overall health, including the health of your nervous system. Their high fiber content aids digestion by promoting regular bowel movements and supporting gut health. Fiber acts like a broom, sweeping and cleaning the intestines and keeping everything moving smoothly. It's a simple yet effective way to enhance digestive health and support vagal function.

Hydration, often underestimated, is another crucial factor in supporting the function of the vagus nerve. Think of water as the oil that keeps your body's engine running smoothly. Staying adequately hydrated ensures that your digestive processes, including those regulated by the vagus nerve, function optimally. Drinking water throughout the day helps maintain the proper balance of fluids in your body, supporting the digestive system's ability to break down food and absorb nutrients. Herbal teas, such as peppermint or ginger tea, can aid digestion and provide a soothing ritual supporting hydration and relaxation.

To further enhance vagal function through nutrition, consider consulting experts for insights on balanced meal planning and recommended supplements. Prebiotics, probiotics, and postbiotics are valuable allies in maintaining a healthy gut microbiome. Prebiotics in foods like garlic and onions feed the beneficial bacteria in your gut. Probiotics, as mentioned earlier, are present in fermented foods and supplements. Postbiotics are the valuable byproducts of probiotic activity, contributing to gut health and immune function. Additionally, fiber supplements and minerals, such as magnesium, can support gastrointestinal function. Magnesium, in particular, can help relax the digestive tract muscles, promoting smoother digestion.

While certain foods support vagal health, others can have the opposite effect. Processed foods high in sugars and unhealthy fats can impair vagal function and disrupt the delicate balance of your gut microbiome. These foods often lead to inflammation, which can affect both your physical and mental well-being. Caffeine, when consumed in excess, can also interfere with the vagus nerve's ability to regulate stress responses and digestion.

Moderation is key, and being mindful of your caffeine intake can help you maintain a balanced nervous system.

Let's look at a sample meal plan to give you a practical idea of incorporating these dietary tips into your daily life. Start your day with gluten-free grains topped with hemp hearts, ground flaxseeds, and various berries for breakfast. This combination provides a rich source of omega-3 fatty acids, fiber, and antioxidants, setting a positive tone for your day. A lunch chicken salad made with avocado mayo, celery, herbs, and pecans with leafy greens and avocado offers healthy fats, protein, and essential nutrients, supporting energy and digestion. Enjoy grilled fish with white sweet potato and steamed vegetables for dinner. This meal is rich in omega-3 fatty acids, fiber, and vitamins, providing a satisfying end to your day while supporting vagal health.

As you explore these dietary tips, remember that small, consistent changes can significantly improve your overall well-being. These choices are not just about what you eat but about nurturing your body and mind, creating a foundation for a healthier, more balanced life. Your diet is a tool that can support your journey toward optimal health, and by focusing on foods that enhance vagus nerve function, you're taking a meaningful step toward lasting wellness.

By recognizing the interconnectedness between diet, digestion, and the vagus nerve, you're empowering yourself with the tools needed for enhanced health. These insights lay the groundwork for a more in-depth exploration of how lifestyle choices can further improve your well-being. Let's continue to build on this foundation. In the next chapter we'll explore how movement and breath can be powerful allies in supporting your vagus nerve and overall health.

Chapter 10: Healing Through Movement, Breath, and Daily Vagal Activation

Picture the rhythmic rise and fall of waves on a tranquil shore. This natural ebb and flow mirrors the gentle exercise of your breath and movement, vital forces that can transform your body's functions. Just as the tides wash over the sand, cleansing and renewing it, intentional movement and breathwork can rejuvenate and balance your nervous system. The vagus nerve, often described as the body's natural pacemaker, thrives on this rhythmic harmony. When nurtured through daily exercises, it can help guide you from a state of heightened stress to one of relaxation and calm.

We have talked throughout this book about how daily vagal stimulation centers on the idea that small, consistent practices can significantly benefit your nervous system. Incorporating these exercises into your daily routine is like tending a garden: with regular care, you cultivate resilience and growth. Morning breathwork rituals serve as a gentle wake-up call for your body and mind, setting a serene tone for the day ahead. As you awaken, deep, diaphragmatic breathing helps activate the parasympathetic nervous system, nudging your body into a state of "rest and digest." Starting each day with intentional breathwork prepares your vagus nerve to handle the day's challenges gracefully and effortlessly. However, there are even more exercises that you can use to create your personalized vagus activation plan.

10.1 Review of Examples of Vagus Activation Exercises

As the day winds down, your plan may include evening relaxation techniques, providing a soothing transition from activity to rest. Engaging in evening relaxation techniques is your opportunity to unwind, signaling to your body that it's time to relax and recharge. Whether it's a calming yoga sequence, a few moments of mindful meditation, or simply focusing on your breath as you lie in bed, these practices help reinforce the day's vagal engagement. They create a bridge from the day's demands to the peace of slumber, nourishing your nervous system as you prepare for restful sleep.

Incorporating additional, specific vagal activation exercises can be simple and effective. Cold exposure therapy, such as a brief cold shower, stimulates the vagus nerve by activating the body's natural stress response and promoting recovery. You can also incorporate cold plunges. This practice can invigorate your body, boosting alertness and resilience. On a different note, humming or chanting creates vibrational stimulation through the vocal cords, engaging the vagus nerve and fostering relaxation. This exercise can be particularly beneficial when stress levels are high as an accessible tool for calming the mind. Gargling, a seemingly mundane task, can activate the throat muscles connected to the vagus nerve, offering another relaxation and stress relief pathway.

Mindfulness techniques further amplify the effects of vagal exercises, enhancing their capacity to promote calm and focus. Mindful meditation, particularly with deep breathing, fosters a profound connection that nurtures both the mind and body. You engage the parasympathetic nervous system by grounding yourself in the present moment and focusing on your breath, inviting peace and clarity. This practice supports vagal tone and cultivates emotional resilience, helping you navigate life's challenges more easily.

Consistency is key to unlocking the full benefits of these practices. Think of it like building a muscle: regular exercise strengthens and fortifies it over time. Similarly, a consistent routine of vagal exercises fosters cumulative benefits for your nervous system, enhancing your ability to manage stress and maintain balance. A daily routine tracker can help you stay committed, allowing you to monitor your progress and celebrate your achievements. By incorporating these practices into your life, you're creating a foundation of well-being that supports your overall health and resilience.

Reflection Exercise:

Take a moment to reflect on your current routines.

Can you make any minor changes to incorporate these vagal exercises into your daily routine?

What would those small changes be?

What would your goals be for these small changes?

Consider setting aside five to ten minutes each morning and evening for breathwork or meditation. Use a journal to track how these practices impact your stress levels and overall well-being. By observing the changes over time, you can gain valuable insights into what works best for you, empowering you to take control of your health and emotional balance.

10.2 Quick Stress Relief Techniques

Stress can ambush us without warning in the fast-paced world we navigate daily. Whether it's an unexpected deadline at work or an emotional trigger from a conversation, stress can quickly escalate, leaving us overwhelmed. In these moments, having immediate stress relief methods readily available can be a lifesaver. Picture yourself sitting at your desk, heart racing as the demands pile up, or standing in the hallway, bracing yourself for a presentation. These scenarios are familiar to many, highlighting the need for quick interventions to calm the storm within. In these high-pressure situations, rapid stress relief techniques come into play, offering a lifeline when you need it most.

Imagine stepping into a busy office, the clatter of keyboards and the murmur of voices a constant backdrop. As the stress builds, your shoulders tighten, and your breath becomes shallow. Progressive muscle relaxation can be your anchor here. This technique involves tensing and then releasing each muscle group from your toes to your head, allowing you to release the tension you are holding in your body. As you focus on the sensation, your mind begins to quiet, your body softens, and a sense of calm washes over you. It's as if you've pressed a reset button, grounding yourself amidst the chaos.

In another scenario, you might find yourself in the car, caught in gridlock traffic, the clock ticking loudly in your mind as you rush to an important meeting. Prayer and/or rapid breathing exercises can be your ally. By saying a quick prayer and practicing quick cycles of inhaling through your nose and exhaling through your mouth, you can disrupt the stress response and bring your nervous system back to equilibrium. This deliberate focus on the words of a prayer and your breath is a bridge, connecting you back to your body and signaling safety to your brain. As you breathe, the tension begins to dissolve, and you navigate the traffic with a newfound patience.

Let's uncover the science behind these quick techniques. When stress strikes, the sympathetic nervous system kicks into high gear, preparing your body for a fight-or-flight response. Your heart rate accelerates, and adrenaline surges through your veins. These rapid techniques activate the parasympathetic nervous system—the calming counterpart to the stress response. By consciously engaging your breath and muscles, you stimulate the vagus nerve, which helps lower heart rate and blood pressure, shifting your body toward a relaxing state. It's like applying brakes on a downhill slope, slowing the momentum and allowing you to regain control.

These quick techniques are not limited to crisis moments. You can integrate them seamlessly into daily life. Picture yourself on a crowded bus or train during your morning commute. Instead of allowing the hustle to overwhelm you, take a moment to practice progressive muscle relaxation or rapid breathing. These simple acts can transform your journey, setting a peaceful tone for your day. Likewise, before stepping onto a stage or entering a room full of expectant eyes, these methods can be your secret weapon against performance anxiety. You anchor yourself in the present by engaging your breath and muscles, ready to face the audience with clarity and confidence.

10.3 Vagal Activation and Resilience

Resilience is like a sturdy tree that bends but doesn't break in the face of a storm. It's the capacity to recover from setbacks, adapt to change, and keep moving forward despite life's challenges. Have you noticed that some people endure constant adversity and still bounce back time after time? This is resilience. Resilience is fundamentally connected to a healthy vagus nerve, crucial in moderating our stress responses and ensuring we recover after adversity. This connection between resilience and stress management is vital, as a well-functioning vagus nerve helps maintain emotional balance and stability. It acts as a buffer, softening the impact of life's inevitable stressors and allowing you to navigate them with grace and tenacity.

Building resilience isn't just about enduring hardship; it's about cultivating strength and adaptability through various practices that enhance vagal tone. Regular physical activity is one such method, as movement stimulates the vagus nerve, promoting cardiovascular health and emotional well-being. Whether it's a brisk walk in the park, a dance class, or a yoga session, physical exercise energizes the body and calms the mind. Furthermore, prayer, practicing gratitude, and positive affirmations can nurture emotional resilience. You create a mental framework that supports positivity and adaptability by focusing on what you appreciate and affirming your strengths and goals. This habitual shift in perspective can profoundly affect your outlook and stress resilience.

Social connections also play a crucial role in bolstering vagal health and resilience. Human beings are inherently social creatures, and the quality of our relationships significantly impacts our well-being. Building supportive relationships and participating in community activities are powerful ways to enhance vagal function and emotional resilience. When you engage with others, share experiences, and offer support, you activate pathways in the brain that foster a sense of safety and belonging. These interactions stimulate the vagus nerve, reinforcing your ability to cope with stress and adversity. Whether joining a church or a local club, attending social gatherings, or simply spending time with loved ones, nurturing your social network is vital to resilience building.

Scientific research underscores the efficacy of vagal activation in enhancing resilience and reducing stress. Studies have shown that individuals with higher vagal tone tend to have more robust stress responses and recover more quickly from stressors. For instance, research on heart rate variability—a measure of vagal tone—shows that individuals with higher variability tend to be more resilient and less prone to stress-related disorders. These findings highlight the vagus nerve's role as a physiological mediator of resilience, supporting the body's ability to maintain homeostasis in the face of challenges. By intentionally engaging in practices stimulating the vagus nerve, you can cultivate this resilience, preparing yourself to handle whatever life throws your way.

The path to resilience is profoundly personal and multifaceted, involving physical and emotional dimensions. It's a journey of self-discovery, growth, and adaptation guided by the body's natural capacity for healing and balance. As a key player in this process, the vagus nerve offers a pathway to resilience through its influence on the autonomic nervous system. Integrating practices that enhance vagal tone into your daily life can strengthen your resilience, empowering you to face life's challenges with confidence and poise.

10.4 Overcoming Skepticism with Results

When considering the practices surrounding vagus nerve stimulation, it's only natural to approach with a healthy dose of skepticism. Many question whether incorporating these exercises is worth their time, especially in our fast-paced world where every minute counts. There is often concern about the commitment required and doubts about the scientific basis supporting these methods. After all, why invest in something if you're uncertain about its effectiveness? These concerns, while understandable, can be addressed by looking at the tangible benefits that others have experienced and the research that supports these practices.

Take Kristi, a busy professional who struggled with persistent brain fog and anxiety. She was initially doubtful about how simple exercises could make a difference. However, after committing to a routine of vagus nerve exercises, she noticed significant improvements in her mental clarity. Her focus sharpened, and she felt more present in her daily tasks. These shifts didn't happen overnight, but her experience highlights the potential impact of consistent practice.

Another example is Daniel, who battled anxiety for years. He was skeptical but decided to try incorporating vagus nerve exercises into his routine. Over time, he found his anxiety levels dropping, and he could manage stress more effectively. These personal stories illustrate the potential of these practices to bring about genuine change, transforming skepticism into belief.

The scientific community has not ignored the vagus nerve's potential. Numerous studies and clinical trials support the efficacy of vagus nerve stimulation. For instance, research has shown that stimulating the vagus nerve can reduce symptoms in conditions like depression and epilepsy. Research is ongoing in numerous areas, like cluster headaches, migraines, strokes, and inflammatory conditions, to name a few. Stimulating the vagus nerve is crucial in regulating the body's stress response and emotional regulation. Studies have demonstrated that consistent stimulation can enhance vagal tone, improving emotional resilience and overall well-being. These findings provide a solid foundation for our practices, reassuring those seeking scientific validation.

It's essential to recognize that what works for one person may not work for another. This is why adopting a trial-and-error approach can be so valuable. You can discover which methods resonate with you by experimenting with different techniques. Some people might find that deep breathing exercises work wonders, while others may benefit more from cold exposure or humming. Also, remember that you may need to use different techniques depending on what your body is telling you it needs. If you awaken and find your voice is a bit hoarse, then utilize some gargling, or if you are having to focus intently on rush hour traffic and starting to feel tense, start praying or singing. It's about finding what fits the situation, your lifestyle, and your needs. There are dozens of books and a great deal of information online about vagus nerve exercises. This personal exploration can help bridge the gap between skepticism and trust, allowing you to tailor your approach to your unique requirements.

By experimenting with these techniques, you open yourself up to learning more about your body and mind. As you begin, you'll notice how different practices affect your mood, stress levels, and overall vitality. This self-discovery process is empowering, encouraging you to take charge of your health and well-being. It's not about rigidly following a prescribed path but about creating your journey of exploration and healing. Opening yourself to trying new things may uncover unexpected benefits that enhance your quality of life. This willingness to explore, adapt, and learn can lead to profound transformations beyond the initial skepticism.

You've explored these practices and their potential impact on your life, but remember that the journey is uniquely yours. There's no one-size-fits-all solution, and that's perfectly okay. Embrace the process with curiosity and an open heart, allowing yourself to learn and grow as you continue through this process. In doing so, you pave the way for personal growth and transformation, leaving skepticism in the rearview mirror. The vagus nerve, with its vast potential for healing and balance, offers a path to greater well-being, and by embracing it, you take an active role in shaping your future. Consider how these practices fit into your life, and don't hesitate to adjust as needed. The key is to remain open to possibilities and trust in your ability to create positive change. As you continue this exploration, know that you are not alone in your journey; countless others have walked this path and found their way to greater well-being, and so can you. As you've discovered, movement, breath, and daily vagal activation are more than physical practices—they are anchors that ground your nervous system and build resilience from the inside out. But the true magic of vagus nerve support happens when these practices become part of a more extensive, integrated lifestyle. In the next chapter, we'll explore how to personalize these strategies, sustain them long-term, and build a supportive ecosystem that allows your health to flourish in every season of life.

Chapter 11: Integrating Practices for Long-Term Health

Imagine stepping into a vibrant garden filled with plants, each requiring a unique blend of sunlight, water, and care to thrive. Like this garden, your health is a complex ecosystem that flourishes when nurtured with personalized attention. In a world where cookie-cutter solutions often fall short, embracing personalized approaches in healthcare can be transformative. Understanding that no two individuals are alike, your journey to wellness should reflect your distinct needs, preferences, and circumstances. This approach ensures that the care you provide for yourself resonates with you and your specific life story, fostering a deeper connection with your body and mind.

11.1 Your Personalized Health Plan

Personalizing your health plan begins with assessing your individual goals and priorities. Take a moment to reflect on what truly matters to you. Perhaps you're seeking balance amidst a hectic schedule or wish to enhance your emotional resilience. Clearly defining what you hope to achieve lays the groundwork for a tailored strategy that aligns with your aspirations.

Consider your lifestyle factors-your daily routine, family commitments, and social interactions. These shape your experience and influence which strategies will serve you best. Acknowledging them enables you to create a plan that flows with your life's natural rhythm, supporting long-term success.

Next, evaluate your current health status. Reflect on your sleep patterns, energy levels, and stress responses-these markers offer a snapshot of your overall well-being, helping you identify areas that require attention. Understanding your vagal tone, the measure of your vagus nerve's health provides insight into your stress response and adaptability. A high vagal tone reflects resilience, while a low tone may highlight areas for growth. Monitoring these indicators gives you a comprehensive view of your health, helping you to make informed, empowered decisions.

You already hold valuable insights if you've completed this book's *Interactive Elements and Reflection Exercises*. To build on this, keep a daily health journal. Track your mood, physical sensations, and stress levels. Journaling encourages mindfulness and helps reveal patterns and triggers over time. Reflecting on these entries, you can identify factors impacting your health, helping to refine your personalized plan further. Like tending a garden, this reflective process enables you to observe, adapt, and refine your approach. Gradually, you'll understand how your body responds in various situations, allowing you to tailor your health plan for optimal outcomes.

> *Reflection Exercise*
>
> *Please take a few minutes to engage in a reflection exercise. Find a quiet space and consider the following prompts:*
>
> *What are your top health priorities?*
>
> *Are there specific areas where you feel stuck or need support?*
>
> *How do your daily habits align with your health goals?*
>
> *Record your thoughts in your journal, allowing the insights to inform your personalized health plan.*

Personalized healthcare offers many benefits, from empowerment and engagement to improved outcomes. By tailoring your approach, you actively participate in your journey, gaining confidence as you align your plan with your body's needs. This method reflects personalized healthcare principles emphasizing your genetic and physiological uniqueness to customize treatments. Your healthcare decisions become increasingly aligned and meaningful with growing awareness and knowledge.

Ultimately, this path transforms your wellness journey into a deeply meaningful experience. It honors your individuality and the complex interplay of factors contributing to your well-being. By embracing personalization, you create a foundation for long-term health and vitality and self-connection.

11.2 Sustaining Practices for Lifelong Benefits

Maintaining health practices long-term can be challenging, feeling like an uphill battle. It's easy to start with enthusiasm, but the real challenge lies in keeping that momentum, which often fades when life throws its inevitable curveballs. You might know the cycle: starting strong, hitting a snag, losing momentum. This cycle is typical. Flexibility becomes your ally. Rather than rigid adherence, aim for balance-showing up consistently while allowing room for adjustments without feeling like you've failed. This perspective shift can keep you on track even when life gets messy.

Long-term success comes from weaving small, meaningful changes into your daily life-one habit at a time. Habit stacking is a powerful technique that we talked about that involves adding new habits to your existing routines. For instance, meditate while your coffee brews or practice mindful breathing on your daily walk. This method leverages your brain's natural pathways, making it easier to incorporate change without feeling overwhelmed.

Setting reminders can also keep you accountable, and an accountability partner- a friend or family member with similar goals and values- can also help. A friend or family member with similar values can support and celebrate your progress and encourage each other during tough times. Regularly reviewing and adjusting your health plan is another vital strategy. Life evolves, and so should your practices. Periodic check-ins help you reassess, preventing stagnation and helping you stay aligned with your changing needs.

Motivation needs both spark and steady fuel. Celebrate small successes and milestones-like a week of consistent journaling or a month of better sleep. Small wins add up, and acknowledging them reinforces positive behavior. Visualization techniques can be powerful and keep you grounded. Picture yourself as vibrant and energized, achieving your goals, and reap the rewards of your hard work. This mental process can make your journey feel tangible and worthwhile. For example, one of my patients, Maria, found success by visualizing her goals daily. She envisioned waking with energy, feeling lighter and more at peace each day. Her consistent visualization helped her stay focused and optimistic even when progress felt slow.

Testimonials from individuals who've maintained their health practice offer insight and inspiration. Take Tyler, for instance. He struggled to maintain a consistent exercise routine, often citing a lack of time as a barrier. Through small changes, such as incorporating short workouts into his lunch breaks, he gradually developed a habit that stuck. Over time, he improved his physical health and found a new sense of accomplishment and resilience. Tyler's story highlights the power of incremental progress, showing that even small steps can lead to significant transformation. This small shift led to improved health and renewed confidence.

Another inspiring example is Kaleigh, who initially struggled with stress management. She began with simple breathing exercises, expanding into yoga and mindfulness practices. Kaleigh's journey was not without setbacks, but she learned to view them as opportunities for growth. Her resilience was fueled by celebrating each small success, reinforcing her commitment to self-care. Today, Kaleigh feels more grounded and capable of handling life's challenges with a calm demeanor.

These examples remind us that sustaining wellness is a dynamic, evolving process. With flexibility and patience, you can adapt and grow. Embrace the journey as an unfolding path, where every step-no matter how small-contributes to meaningful change.

11.3 Building a Supportive Community

Imagine being part of a group where you feel understood, valued, and inspired. Being involved in a group is the essence of a supportive community, a powerful force in any health journey. Having a network of people who share similar goals can encourage you to keep moving forward. In a community, you find a safe space to share your experiences, learn from others, and celebrate victories together. This sense of belonging enhances motivation and accountability as you become part of a collective effort toward well-being. Engaging in group activities fosters camaraderie, making maintaining health practices more enjoyable and less isolating.

To build and engage with a supportive community, seek out local wellness groups or online forums that align with your interests and needs. Many communities offer group workshops and events focused on health and wellness, providing opportunities to connect with like-minded individuals. Participating in these gatherings broadens your perspective and opens the door to new friendships and collaborations. Online platforms can be equally valuable, offering a virtual space to share insights, ask questions, and receive guidance from people worldwide. These connections can be a source of strength when facing challenges, reminding you that you're not alone in your efforts.

The impact of social support on health outcomes is well-documented. Research indicates that individuals with strong community ties tend to experience improved mental health and increased adherence to healthy practices. Being part of a community can help reduce feelings of isolation and encourage positive behaviors, ultimately leading to improved overall well-being. Studies have shown that individuals participating in various group settings are more likely to adhere to their health routines, thanks to the added accountability and encouragement. This collective effort can yield meaningful changes as members inspire one another to strive for their best.

Creating a positive and inclusive community environment requires intentional effort. Encourage open communication and empathy, allowing everyone to feel heard and respected. By fostering an atmosphere of understanding, you help build trust and solidarity among members. Regular meetups or virtual check-ins can strengthen these bonds, providing consistent opportunities for connection and support. Organizing these in-person or online gatherings helps maintain momentum and keeps the community engaged. Encourage members to share their stories, challenges, and triumphs, creating a tapestry of experiences that enriches the group. This sharing forms the backbone of a supportive community where everyone learns and grows together.

Building and nurturing a community can transform your health journey. It provides a sense of belonging and purpose, reminding you of the power of collective strength. Whether through local groups or virtual spaces, these connections become a vital resource, offering encouragement and insight when needed. By engaging with others who share your goals, you create a network of support that reinforces your commitment to health and well-being. This sense of community becomes a source of resilience, empowering you to face challenges confidently and gracefully.

Finding and fostering community is more important than ever in an increasingly disconnected world. It reminds us of our shared humanity and the impact we can have on each other's lives. As you continue on your path to health, consider the role that community can play in your journey. Embrace the opportunities to connect, share, and learn from those around you, knowing that together, you can achieve more than you ever thought possible.

11.4 Embracing a Holistic Health Mindset

Imagine viewing health not as isolated parts but as a dynamic, interconnected system where mind, body, and spirit are in constant dialogue. This holistic health mindset perspective encourages us to see beyond symptoms, focusing instead on the whole person. It's about recognizing that emotional well-being, physical health, and spiritual fulfillment are deeply intertwined. Consider your health as a symphony, where each aspect contributes to the harmony of the whole. Embracing this mindset invites adaptability in health practices, encouraging us to flow with life's changes rather than resist them. This adaptability is crucial because our needs evolve and are influenced by life's unpredictable nature. By seeing health as an evolving entity, we can better navigate the shifts and turns that come our way.

The benefits of a holistic approach to health are profound. By considering the whole person, we unlock enhanced emotional resilience, enabling us to weather life's storms more easily. It's not just about coping with stress but thriving amidst it, finding strength in vulnerability. Physical health also improves through integrated practices that harmonize with our unique rhythms. Imagine a life where exercise, nutrition, mindfulness, and social connections are not separate activities but threads woven into the fabric of daily living. This integration fosters a sense of balance and fulfillment, where each action supports the others, creating a life of vitality and purpose.

Cultivating a holistic health mindset begins with mindfulness and self-awareness. Taking the time to tune into your thoughts, feelings, and bodily sensations fosters a deeper connection with yourself. The many simple practices discussed throughout this book, such as meditation, breathwork, or even a quiet walk in nature, can anchor you in the present moment, offering clarity and insight. This awareness becomes the foundation for exploring many complementary therapies and practices that resonate with you. These might include acupuncture, yoga, Qigong, Tai Chi, homeopathy, or herbal medicine, offering unique pathways to balance and healing. As you explore, maintain an openness to new ideas and experiences, allowing curiosity to guide your journey. This openness fosters growth, broadening your understanding of health and your connection to it.

Consider the story of Emma, who found herself struggling with chronic stress and fatigue. Traditional treatments offered little relief, prompting her to explore a holistic approach. She integrated mindfulness meditation into her routine, began practicing yoga, and sought guidance from a Naturopathic Doctor. Over time, Emma noticed a profound shift in her well-being. Her stress levels decreased, her energy improved, and she felt more connected to herself and others. This transformation wasn't about finding a quick fix but embracing a lifestyle that honored her entire being. Emma's narrative illustrates the potential for healing and happiness when we view health holistically.

Similarly, Nick's journey highlights the power of an integrated approach. Battling digestive issues for years, he turned to a combination of dietary changes, stress management techniques, and acupuncture. As he adopted this comprehensive strategy, Nick experienced a significant reduction in symptoms and increased overall vitality. He learned to listen to his body's signals, adapting his practices to meet changing needs. For Nick, holistic health became a way of life, offering a sense of balance and fulfillment he had long sought.

These examples underscore the potential of a holistic health mindset to transform lives. By honoring the interconnectedness of mind, body, and spirit, we create a foundation for lasting well-being. This mindset invites us to see health not as a destination but as an ongoing process of discovery and growth. As we continue to explore this expansive view of health, we open ourselves to new possibilities and insights, enriching our lives in ways we never imagined.

By embracing a holistic health mindset, we embark on the road of continuous learning and adaptation. This journey is not without challenges, but we draw closer to a life of balance, resilience, and fulfillment with each mile. Let this mindset guide us as we move forward, nourishing our connection to ourselves and the world around us. In doing so, we cultivate a life of vitality and purpose that honors the whole person and celebrates the beauty of being truly alive. You've gathered a powerful collection of tools, insights, and practices that honor your unique path to healing and vitality. From tuning into your body to building community and embracing a holistic mindset, you are equipped to move forward with intention and confidence. In the conclusion, we'll reflect on the journey we've taken together and offer final thoughts to inspire and empower you as you continue nurturing your vagus nerve—and your well-being—for the road ahead.

Final Words Before the Conclusion

You've gathered powerful tools-rooted in science but nourished by self-awareness and compassion. From tracking your progress to building a meaningful community, you're creating a life that supports your healing from the inside out.

In the conclusion, we'll take a moment to reflect on everything you've learned and share a few final insights to carry with you on the journey ahead.

YOUR REVIEW CAN HELP SOMEONE HEAL

A Small Act of Kindness Can Make a Big Difference

"I've learned that people will forget what you said, people will forget what you did, but people will never forget how you made them feel." – Maya Angelou

When we give something—our time, our care, or even just a kind word—we often help someone more than we realize. And sometimes, that simple act can help someone feel less alone, more hopeful, and ready to take the next step.

If this book helped you understand your body better, feel more connected, or gave you tools to feel more calm and healthy, would you consider helping someone else who's searching for those same things?

That's the power of leaving a review.

Many people don't know where to begin when they feel overwhelmed by pain, stress, or health problems. A review like yours might be the light they need to see a way forward and start their healing journey.

I wrote this book to make the science of the vagus nerve simple and easy to understand so more people could regain their health and feel more in control of their bodies and minds. But to reach more people, I need your help.

Most people choose a book based on what other readers say. Your voice matters.

Leaving a review is quick, free, and means so much. Your few words might help:

- One more mom or dad finally **sleep** better at night.
- One more person with **anxiety** find a new way to feel calm.
- One more teen understand their **emotions**.

- One more person with **stomach pain** realize it's not "all in their head."
- One more friend begin their **journey toward real healing.**

If that sounds like something you'd love to be a part of, just scan the QR code below or click the link to leave a review:

https://www.amazon.com/review/review-your-purchases/?asin=1968147012

Thank you, truly, from the bottom of my heart.

Your kindness keeps this mission moving.

With deep gratitude,

Dr. Kerri L. Jones, N.M.D.

Remember, if you have enjoyed this book, be sure get my next book in this series, ***Unleash Your Vagus Nerve Superhighway Potential: Explore Holistic Therapies for Nervous System Repair and Balance, Emotional Resilience, Immune Support, and Vital Energy Restoration.*** This book discusses my specific recommendations and prescriptions to help you formulate your own plan to heal your life!

Conclusion

As we wrap up this journey through the wonders of the vagus nerve, I invite you to reflect on the profound insights we've explored together. We've uncovered how this incredible nerve serves as a vital link between the brain and body-regulating our physical health, emotional well-being, and capacity for resilience.

A key takeaway is the **power of awareness**. By understanding how the vagus nerve functions and how imbalances can affect our health, we gain the ability to make meaningful changes. Simple, consistent practices like deep breathing, mindfulness, and cold exposure can significantly improve vagal tone and enhance your well-being. When these tools become part of your daily rhythm, they empower lasting transformation.

Equally important is learning to **listen to your body**. The vagus nerve constantly sends messages that can guide you toward balance and healing-if you're willing to tune in. Whether it's resting when overwhelmed, choosing nourishing foods, or nurturing healthy relationships, honoring your body's wisdom leads to greater ease and vitality.

This journey is deeply personal. Start small. Trust your intuition. Be curious and compassionate with yourself as you explore what supports your unique healing path. Progress may come in waves, but every step you take builds resilience and deepens your connection with yourself.

I speak not only as a doctor but as someone who has walked this path. By applying the strategies in this book, I've experienced firsthand how small changes can ripple into a life of greater balance, clarity, and joy. I believe the same is possible for you.

Thank you for allowing me to be a part of your healing journey. Your willingness to learn, grow, and take ownership of your health is truly inspiring. Remember, you are the author of your story-and the vagus nerve is a powerful ally in guiding you toward a life of greater health, peace, and purpose.

If you're ready to dive even deeper, I invite you to explore my upcoming book, ***The Naturopathic Doctor's Vagus Nerve Superhighway Code: Complete Holistic Medicine Protocols for Nervous System Repair, Emotional Healing, Immune Resilience, and Vital Energy Restoration.*** This comprehensive guide shares my most effective naturopathic treatments and protocols—from targeted nutrition and herbal remedies to lifestyle therapies-to help you restore balance, overcome burnout, and reclaim vibrant energy and health.

You've taken a powerful step forward. Let your vagus nerve be your compass as you continue creating the vibrant, empowered life you deserve.

References

- **Allied Services.** (2020). *The vagus nerve: Your secret weapon in fighting stress.* Retrieved March 26, 2025, from https://www.allied-services.org/news/2020/june/the-vagus-nerve-your-secret-weapon-in-fighting-s/

- **American Heart Association.** (2024). *Vagus nerve stimulation and inflammation in cardiovascular disease. Journal of the American Heart Association, 13*(5), e030539. https://doi.org/10.1161/JAHA.123.030539

- **Ballard, J.** (n.d.). *How to activate the vagus nerve for emotional balance and inner calm.* Retrieved March 26, 2025, from https://ballard-phd.com/how-to-activate-the-vagus-nerve-for-emotional-balance-and-inner-calm/

- **Beekwilder, J., & Beems, T.** (2010). Vagus nerve stimulation in partial epilepsy: Clinical results and mechanisms of action. *European Neurology, 63*(3), 148–153. https://doi.org/10.1159/000276366

- **Bioelectronic Medicine.** (2022). *Vagus nerve stimulation and inflammation: Expanding the therapeutic spectrum. Bioelectronic Medicine, 8,* 14. https://doi.org/10.1186/s42234-022-00100-3

- **BMC Medicine.** (2023). *Multimodal non-invasive non-pharmacological therapies for chronic pain. BMC Medicine, 21,* 147. htt ps://doi.org/10.1186/s12916-023-03076-2

- **Breit, S., Kupferberg, A., Rogler, G., & Hasler, G.** (2018). Vagus nerve as modulator of the brain–gut axis in psychiatric and inflammatory disorders. *Frontiers in Psychiatry, 9*, 44. https://doi.org/10.3389/fpsyt.2018.00044
- **Centers for Medicare & Medicaid Services.** (n.d.). *Vagus nerve stimulation (VNS) for treatment resistant depression*. Retrieved March 26, 2025, from https://www.cms.gov/medicare/coverage/evidence/vagus-nerve-stimulation
- **Cleveland Clinic.** (n.d.). *Vagus nerve: What it is, function, location & conditions*. Retrieved March 26, 2025, from https://my.clevelandclinic.org/health/body/22279-vagus-nerve
- **Clapp, M., Aurora, N., Herrera, L., Bhatia, M., Wilen, E., & Wakefield, S.** (2017). Gut microbiota's effect on mental health: The gut-brain axis. *Clinical Practice, 7*(4), 987. https://doi.org/10.4081/cp.2017.987
- **Colorado Pain Care.** (n.d.). *Benefits of personalized healthcare*. Retrieved March 26, 2025, from http://coloradopaincare.com/benefits-of-personalized-healthcare/
- **Cindy Jakubiec, D. C.** (n.d.). *10 ways to stimulate your vagus nerve (+ why it's important)*. Retrieved March 26, 2025, from https://drcindyjakubiec.com/10-ways-to-stimulate-your-vagus-nerve-why-its-important/
- **Everyday Health.** (n.d.). *7 ways to stimulate your vagus nerve and why it matters*. Retrieved March 26, 2025, from https://www.everydayhealth.com/neurology/ways-to-stimulate-your-vagus-nerve-and-why-it-matters/

- **Frontiers in Psychiatry.** (2018). *Vagus nerve as modulator of the brain–gut axis in psychiatric and inflammatory disorders. Frontiers in Psychiatry, 9*, 44. https://www.frontiersin.org/journals/psychiatry/articles/10.3389/fpsyt.2018.00044/full

- **Feinstein Institutes for Medical Research.** (2020). *Vagus nerve stimulation boosts immunity*. Retrieved March 26, 2025, from https://feinstein.northwell.edu/news/the-latest/vagus-nerve-spleen-boost-immunity

- **Frangos, E., & Komisaruk, B. R.** (2017). Accessing the vagus nerve through the auricular branch: Stimulation using non-invasive devices. *Frontiers in Neuroscience, 11*, 557. https://doi.org/10.3389/fnins.2017.00557

- **Gastro SB.** (n.d.). *The vagus nerve and digestion... What's the connection?* Retrieved March 26, 2025, from https://www.gastrosb.com/the-vagus-nerve-and-digestion-whats-the-connection

- **Gidron, Y., Deschepper, R., De Couck, M., Thayer, J. F., & Velkeniers, B.** (2018). The vagus nerve and the inflammatory reflex—linking immunity and emotions. *Journal of Neuroimmunology, 315*, 7–15. https://doi.org/10.1016/j.jneuroim.2017.11.014

- **Hays, S. A.** (2016). Targeting plasticity with vagus nerve stimulation to treat neurological disease. *Progress in Brain Research, 207*, 275–299. https://doi.org/10.1016/bs.pbr.2016.04.009

- **Health.com.** (n.d.). *Holistic health: A guide to better health and well-being*. Retrieved March 26, 2025, from https://www.health.com/holistic-health-8652522

- **IntechOpen.** (2023). *Neurotransmitters of autonomic nervous system*. Retrieved March 26, 2025, from https://www.intechop

en.com/chapters/88176

- **Ivory Plains Recovery.** (n.d.). *How habit stacking improves wellness*. Retrieved March 26, 2025, from https://ivoryplainsrecovery.com/blog/how-habit-stacking-improves-wellness/

- **Johns Hopkins Medicine.** (n.d.). *Role of vagus nerve stimulation in the treatment of chronic pain*. Retrieved March 26, 2025, from https://www.hopkinsmedicine.org/neurology_neurosurgery/centers_clinics/pain_center/treatments/vagus_nerve_stimulation.html

- **Kenhub.** (n.d.). *Vagus nerve: Anatomy, function, and branches*. Retrieved March 26, 2025, from https://www.kenhub.com/en/library/anatomy/the-vagus-nerve

- **Koopman, F. A., & Tak, P. P.** (2022). Vagus nerve stimulation and inflammation: Expanding the therapeutic spectrum. *Bioelectronic Medicine, 8*, 14. https://doi.org/10.1186/s42234-022-00100-3

- **Lamb, D. G., Porges, S. W., Lewis, G. F., & Williamson, J. B.** (2017). Non-invasive vagal nerve stimulation effects on hyperarousal and autonomic state in patients with posttraumatic stress disorder. *Frontiers in Psychiatry, 8*, 44. https://doi.org/10.3389/fpsyt.2017.00044

- **LivaNova.** (n.d.). *Testimonials | VNS therapy*. Retrieved March 26, 2025, from https://www.livanova.com/epilepsy-vnstherapy/en-us/testimonials

- **Massachusetts General Hospital.** (n.d.). *The vagus nerve: A key player in your health and well-being*. Retrieved March 26, 2025, from https://www.massgeneral.org/news/article/vagus-nerve

- **NCBI.** (2023). *Recognizing the role of the vagus nerve in depression from inflammation to treatment. Frontiers in Psychiatry*. https://pmc.ncbi.nlm.nih.gov/articles/PMC9685564/
- **NCBI Bookshelf.** (2022). *Social support - Health promotion in health care*. In *StatPearls*. https://www.ncbi.nlm.nih.gov/books/NBK585650/
- **Pardo, J. V., Sheikh, S. A., Kuskowski, M. A., Surerus-Johnson, C., Hagen, M. C., Lee, J. T., & Adson, D. E.** (2007). Functional magnetic resonance imaging during vagus nerve stimulation in epilepsy. *Epilepsy & Behavior, 10*(3), 479–485. https://doi.org/10.1016/j.yebeh.2006.12.005
- **Polyvagal Institute.** (n.d.). *What is polyvagal theory?* Retrieved March 26, 2025, from https://www.polyvagalinstitute.org/whatispolyvagaltheory
- **Porges, S. W.** (1995). Vagal tone and the physiological regulation of emotion. *Monographs of the Society for Research in Child Development, 59*(2–3), 167–186. https://doi.org/10.1111/j.1540-5834.1994.tb01283.x
- **Pyramid Healthcare.** (n.d.). *Treating trauma with polyvagal theory*. Retrieved March 26, 2025, from https://www.pyramid-healthcare.com/treating-trauma-with-polyvagal-theory/
- **Sacred Path Holistic Therapy.** (n.d.). *Polyvagal self-assessment*. Retrieved March 26, 2025, from https://sacredpathholistictherapy.com/polyvagal-assessment/
- **Stephen Porges.** (n.d.). *Stephen W. Porges, PhD | Polyvagal theory*. Retrieved March 26, 2025, from https://www.stephenporges.com/

- **StatPearls.** (2023). *Neuroanatomy, cranial nerve 10 (vagus nerve).* In *StatPearls.* StatPearls Publishing. https://www.ncbi.nlm.nih.gov/books/NBK537171/

- **Top Doctors.** (n.d.). *Vagus nerve dysfunction: Its main causes and symptoms.* Retrieved March 26, 2025, from https://www.topdoctors.co.uk/medical-articles/vagus-nerve-dysfunction-what-is-it-and-what-are-the-main-symptoms

- **Verywell Mind.** (2023). *How stress affects the vagus nerve.* Retrieved March 26, 2025, from https://www.verywellmind.com/how-stress-affects-the-vagus-nerve-6740155

- **Wikipedia contributors.** (n.d.). *Auricular branch of vagus nerve. Wikipedia.* Retrieved March 26, 2025, from https://en.wikipedia.org/wiki/Auricular_branch_of_vagus_nerve

- **Wisemind Nutrition.** (n.d.). *Linking the vagus nerve and gut health.* Retrieved March 26, 2025, from https://wisemindnutrition.com/blog/linking-vagus-nerve-gut-health

- **Yogaru.** (n.d.). *Evening wind down.* Retrieved March 26, 2025, from https://www.yogaru.ie/pause/evening-wind-down

Made in United States
Troutdale, OR
06/12/2026

50010460R00086